Staphylococcal Infections - Recent Advances and Perspectives

Edited by Jaime Bustos-Martínez and Juan José Valdez-Alarcón

Published in London, United Kingdom

Staphylococcal Infections - Recent Advances and Perspectives
http://dx.doi.org/10.5772/intechopen.100798
Edited by Jaime Bustos-Martínez and Juan José Valdez-Alarcón

Contributors
Liang Wang, Xue-Di Zhang, Bin Gu, Muhammad Usman, Jia-Wei Tang, Zheng-Kang Li, Xin-Qiang Zhang, Jia-Wei Yan, Songul Cetik Yildiz, Miguel Ángel Ortíz Gil, Monica Irasu Cardona Alvarado, Jaime Bustos-Martínez, Samuel González-García, Juan José Valdez-Alarcón, Aida Hamdan-Partida, Anaíd Bustos-Hamdan, František Zigo, Zuzana Farkašová, Ibrahim Farag Mohammed Rehan, Ahmed Sayed-Ahmed, Asdren Zajmi, Mohammed A. M. Alhoot, Fathimath Shiranee, Sairah Abdul Karim, Shirley Gee Hoon Tang, Abdalmohaimen Suood, Iman Mahdi, Mahmood Saleh, Enitan Omobolanle Adesanya, Akingbolabo Daniel Ogunlakin

First published in London, United Kingdom, 2023 by IntechOpen
IntechOpen is the global imprint of INTECHOPEN LIMITED, registered in England and Wales, registration number: 11086078, 5 Princes Gate Court, London, SW7 2QJ, United Kingdom
Printed in Croatia

British Library Cataloguing-in-Publication Data
A catalogue record for this book is available from the British Library

Additional hard and PDF copies can be obtained from orders@intechopen.com

Staphylococcal Infections - Recent Advances and Perspectives
Edited by Jaime Bustos-Martínez and Juan José Valdez-Alarcón
p. cm.

This title is part of the Infectious Diseases Book Series, Volume 17
Topic: Bacterial Infectious Diseases
Series Editor: Alfonso J. Rodriguez-Morales
Topic Editors: Tomas Jarzembowski and Katarzyna Garbacz

Print ISBN 978-1-83769-985-8
Online ISBN 978-1-83768-206-5
eBook (PDF) ISBN 978-1-83768-207-2
ISSN 2631-6188

For EU product safety concerns:
IN TECH d.o.o., Prolaz Marije Krucifikse Kozulić 3, 51000 Rijeka, Croatia,
info@intechopen.com or visit our website at intechopen.com.

IntechOpen Book Series
Infectious Diseases
Volume 17

Aims and Scope of the Series

This series will provide a comprehensive overview of recent research trends in various Infectious Diseases (as per the most recent Baltimore classification). Topics will include general overviews of infections, immunopathology, diagnosis, treatment, epidemiology, etiology, and current clinical recommendations for managing infectious diseases. Ongoing issues, recent advances, and future diagnostic approaches and therapeutic strategies will also be discussed. This book series will focus on various aspects and properties of infectious diseases whose deep understanding is essential for safeguarding the human race from losing resources and economies due to pathogens.

Meet the Series Editor

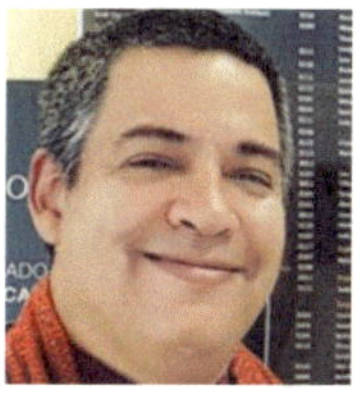

Dr. Rodriguez-Morales is an expert in tropical and emerging diseases, particularly zoonotic and vector-borne diseases (especially arboviral diseases). He is the president of the Travel Medicine Committee of the Pan-American Infectious Diseases Association (API), as well as the president of the Colombian Association of Infectious Diseases (ACIN). He is a member of the Committee on Tropical Medicine, Zoonoses, and Travel Medicine of ACIN. He is a vice-president of the Latin American Society for Travel Medicine (SLAMVI) and a Member of the Council of the International Society for Infectious Diseases (ISID). Since 2014, he has been recognized as a Senior Researcher, at the Ministry of Science of Colombia. He is a professor at the Faculty of Medicine of the Fundacion Universitaria Autonoma de las Americas, in Pereira, Risaralda, Colombia. He is an External Professor, Master in Research on Tropical Medicine and International Health, Universitat de Barcelona, Spain. He is also a professor at the Master in Clinical Epidemiology and Biostatistics, Universidad Científica del Sur, Lima, Peru. In 2021 he has been awarded the "Raul Isturiz Award" Medal of the API. Also, in 2021, he was awarded with the "Jose Felix Patiño" Asclepius Staff Medal of the Colombian Medical College, due to his scientific contributions to COVID-19 during the pandemic. He is currently the Editor in Chief of the journal Travel Medicine and Infectious Diseases. His Scopus H index is 47 (Google Scholar H index, 68).

Meet the Volume Editors

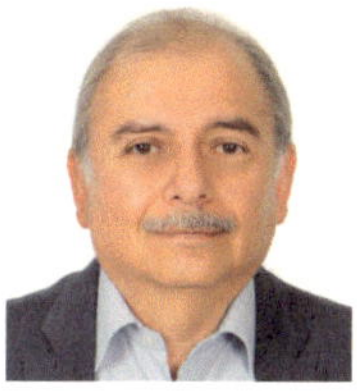

Dr. Jaime Bustos-Martínez is a Research Professor at the Universidad Autónoma Metropolitana-Xochimilco, in Mexico City, Mexico. He has a degree in biological pharmaceutical chemistry, an MSc in biochemical sciences and a Ph.D. in biomedical sciences. For more than 20 years he has been studying virulence factors, molecular epidemiology and nanoparticles against *Staphylococcus aureus*. His studies have been published in several articles in indexed journals and have been presented in international forums. His publications include several textbook chapters and he is a reviewer for multiple journals. He is part of Mexico's National System of Researchers.

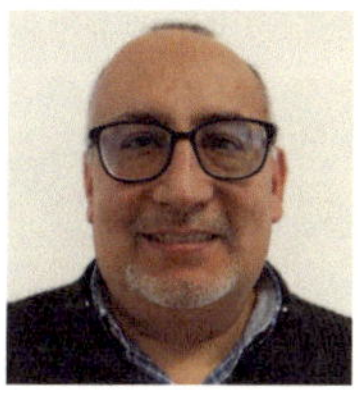

Dr. Juan José Valdez-Alarcón is a Research Professor at the Faculty of Veterinary Medicine and Animal Production in the Multidisciplinary Center for Studies in Biotechnology at the Universidad Michoacana de San Nicolás de Hidalgo, Michoacán, Mexico. A microbiologist with a Ph.D. in biotechnology, his research focus is molecular epidemiology and biotechnology approaches to the study and control of bacterial diseases in animals. He has published more than 60 research papers in national and international scientific journals and nine book chapters. He has also been a member of advisory committees for national and international scientific meetings, a reviewer of microbiology topics for well-recognized scientific journals, and is currently Coordinator of the Animal Microbiology Network of the Microbial and Invertebrates Genetic Resources Subcommittee of the Agricultural and Rural Development Secretariat in Mexico.

Contents

Preface

Staphylococci is a bacterial genus with high pathogenic potential for both humans and animals, especially dairy animals. In this broad group of bacteria, 85 species and 30 subspecies have currently been reported, generally divided into two large groups: coagulase positive (CPS) and coagulase negative (CNS) staphylococci.

Within the coagulase positive group is *Staphylococcus aureus,* which is the main pathogen for humans and livestock and companion animals; the main coagulase negative strain is *S. epidermidis*. However, other species have caused infections and should not be ignored. A high percentage of people carry this microorganism in different parts of the body, mainly in the nose; data increasingly points to a high percentage of carriers also in the pharynx.

S. aureus can colonize and behave as a commensal; the colonization process is a fundamental part of the life cycle of the bacteria. Under certain circumstances, including environmental, bacterial and host factors, they can produce a wide variety of infections ranging from mild to fatal. The severity of *S. aureus* infections is mainly due to the existence of antibiotic-resistant strains, especially methicillin-resistant *S. aureus* (MRSA) strains, which appeared within a few years of the introduction of methicillin replacing penicillin, to which there was already a high percentage of resistant strains, for the treatment of this bacterium.

At first these strains were only found in hospital environments, mainly causing nosocomial infections, and were called hospital-acquired MRSA (HA-MRSA) strains. However, since the 1990s they have moved into the community, causing infections in people who had not been in a hospital environment. The WHO issued a global alert for the prevention and combat of the new strains, which became known as community-acquired MRSA (CA-MRSA). These strains, however, have managed to return to hospitals, now causing new infections in hospitals as well.

Years after the appearance of CA-MRSA strains, MRSA strains were found in livestock workers, giving rise to the group of MRSA strains acquired from livestock (LA-MRSA). This indicates that *S. aureus* strains present in animals can be passed to humans and vice versa.

All of this speaks to the ongoing evolutionary dynamics of staphylococci, especially *S. aureus*.

What is it that makes this microorganism so pathogenic and able to adapt to changes in the host and the environment? How can we determine the presence of staphylococci and their virulence factors? What new treatments are there to combat this microorganism? These are some of the questions that this book seeks to answer.

The first section brings together several chapters referring to colonization by *Staphylococcus aureus* and the factors involved in the process. The second section concerns the epidemiology and pathogenesis of *S. aureus*. The third section is related to the diagnosis of the bacteria and its virulence factors. The last section explores new compounds with antibacterial activity against staphylococci.

In the first section, "*Staphylococcus aureus* and Methicillin Resistant *Staphylococcus aureus* (MRSA) Carriage and Infections", reviews *S. aureus* and MRSA strains in relation to their carriage in humans, their pathogenesis, their resistance to antibiotics, the diseases they cause and their treatment. "Multidrug-Resistant *Staphylococcus aureus as* Coloniser in Healthy Individuals" analyzes the relationship between colonization by *S. aureus* and the possibility of causing disease in carriers through carrying a bacterium that can be dangerous due to its pathogenic properties and their resistance to antibiotics.

The second section contains two chapters on the epidemiology and pathogenesis of *S. aureus*. The colonization of *S. aureus,* the initial process through which this microorganism can produce a disease or persist for a long time in the host is described in "Main Factors of *Staphylococcus aureus* Associated with the Interaction to the Cells for Their Colonization and Persistence". This chapter also discusses the molecules involved in the adhesion of the bacteria to the host cells and their regulation mechanism, as well as biofilm formation, an important part of the colonization process. The evolution of the *S. aureus* strains produces variations in the colonization of the population, leading to changes at the epidemiological level. An example case is described in "The Molecular Epidemiological Study of MRSA in Mexico". Such epidemiological studies contribute to the understanding and development of possible control measures for this microorganism.

Section three consists of two chapters related to diagnosis, an important part of the fight against staphylococci and an essential process in the detection and control of infections they cause. "Recent Progress in the Diagnosis of *Staphylococcus* in Clinical Settings" reviews different methods to detect these microorganisms, from conventional microbiological methods, through molecular methods to the advanced technique of surface-enhanced Raman spectroscopy (SERS). The significance of staphylococcal infections for the livestock sector, especially dairy animals, is covered in "Occurrence of Mastitis in Dairy Herds and the Detection of Virulence Factors in Staphylococci", which describes coagulase negative and methicillin-resistant staphylococcal mastitis infections.

The ability of staphylococci to resist multiple antibiotics enhances their pathogenic capacity, which is why new substances that can eliminate these bacteria are needed. The search for new compounds with antibacterial activity against staphylococci is presented in Section four. The use of silver and copper nanoparticles as an alternative to combat staphylococci is discussed in "The Ability of Some Inorganic Nanoparticles to Inhibit Some *Staphylococcus* spp.". The second chapter of this section, "Potential Use of African Botanicals and Other Compounds in the Treatment of Methicillin-Resistant *Staphylococcus aureus* Infections", analyzes the use of various active substances from medicinal plants that have shown antibacterial action against staphylococci and especially against MRSA strains.

We hope readers will enjoy this book and find information and recent advances relevant to the study of colonization, diagnosis, and treatment of staphylococci, and especially of *S. aureus* and MRSA strains.

Dr. Jaime Bustos-Martínez
Department of Health Care,
Autonomous Metropolitan University-Xochimilco,
Mexico City, Mexico

Dr. Juan José Valdez-Alarcón
Multidisciplinary Center for Studies in Biotechnology,
Faculty of Veterinary Medicine and Zootechnics,
Universidad Michoacana de San Nicolás de Hidalgo,
Michoacán, Mexico

Section 1

Colonization

Chapter 1

Staphylococcus aureus and Methicillin Resistant *Staphylococcus aureus* (MRSA) Carriage and Infections

Songul Cetik Yildiz

Abstract

Staphylococcus aureus is among the most common opportunistic infections worldwide, as it is found as part of the flora in many parts of the body. *S. aureus* is the leading cause of nosocomial infections with its ability to rapidly colonize the infected area, high virulence, rapid adaptation to environmental conditions, and the ability to develop very fast and effective resistance even to new generation antibiotics. Methicillin-resistant *Staphylococcus aureus* (MRSA), first identified in the 1960s, is one of the most successful modern pathogens, becoming an important factor in hospitals in the 1980s. MRSA is an important factor, especially in hospitalized patients and healthcare-associated infections. Patients colonized with *S. aureus* and MRSA are at risk for community-acquired infections. It is critical that multidrug resistance reduces treatment options in MRSA infections and MRSA strains. These microorganisms have been the subject of research for years as they spread and become resistant in both social and medical settings and cause great morbidity and mortality. With the rapid spread of resistance among bacteria, antibiotic resistance has increased the cost of health care, and this has become the factor limiting the production of new antibiotics.

Keywords: *Staphylococcus aureus*, MRSA, infections, antibiotic resistance

1. Introduction

Staphylococcus aureus is the most virulent member of the staphylococcal species. The development of infection depends on the balance between the virulence of the microorganism and the host defence system. *S. aureus* is a versatile, highly adaptive pathogen and is ubiquitous, capable of colonizing the skin and mucous membranes of the anterior nostrils, gastrointestinal tract, perineum, genitourinary tract, and pharynx. *S. aureus* can cause community-acquired and healthcare-associated infections with high morbidity and mortality. It is most commonly isolated from wound infections, urinary tract infections, pneumonia, septic arthritis, osteomyelitis, endocarditis and sepsis, skin and soft tissue infections, bloodstream infections, and hospital-acquired postoperative wound infections.

S. aureus, which is an opportunistic pathogen, has been one of the most frequently isolated pathogens, both from the hospital and from the community, which can lead to more serious infections in the presence of suitable conditions. For the first time in the 1940s, when an *S. aureus* strain developed resistance to penicillin, the development of antibiotic resistance in *S. aureus* was recognized. Methicillin-resistant *S. aureus* (MRSA), which is also virulent, also shows multidrug resistance and has all the pathogenic properties of *S. aureus* strains. The feature that provides methicillin resistance in *S. aureus* is associated with PBP2a, which is encoded by the *mecA* gene complex. Detection of *mecA* gene by molecular methods is the gold standard in the detection of methicillin resistance. Accurate detection of methicillin resistance as soon as possible is of great importance in the control, treatment and selection of the right antibiotic for MRSA infections. Attempts to develop a vaccine for MRSA have so far been unsuccessful. Finally, in 2018, the Pfizer multi-antigen vaccine phase IIb trial (2018) was also stopped on the grounds that it was useless.

Treatment of bacterial infections is a major problem due to the development of resistance. The discovery and development of new drugs are of great importance in order to overcome this problem, which significantly weakens the clinical effectiveness of traditional antibiotics. In this review, we aimed to summarize the extensive literature on the epidemiology, transmission, genetic diversity, evolution, surveillance, and treatment of MRSA by providing an overview of basic and clinical MRSA research.

2. *Staphylococcus aureus*

Gram-positive, non-motile, cocci-shaped, coagulase-positive *S. aureus* is the most clinically important species among 52 species and 28 subspecies in the *Staphylococcus* [1]. The stability and worldwide spread of this pathogen are due to its ability to rapidly acquire and lose determinants of resistance and virulence from other members of the *Staphylococcus* [2]. *S. aureus* is a really hardy bacterium. It is resistant to drying out and it can survive on dry surfaces for a long time. It can survive even at high salt concentrations, providing a basis for selection of the growth medium from other bacteria. They may contain genes responsible for their virulence and resistance to various antibiotics in their chromosomes.

2.1 Pathogenesis of *S. aureus*

Staphylococci were first described by Robert Koch in 1878 and were reported to cause disease in mice by Alexander Ogston in 1881 [3]. *S. aureus*, the most pathogenic member of staphylococci, is the cause of many life-threatening diseases such as superficial skin abscess, food poisoning, bacteremia, necrotic pneumonia in children and endocarditis [4]. The ability of *S. aureus* to infect is realized by the colonization of the bacteria into the host cells. After birth, the umbilical region, perineal region, nose, and gastrointestinal tract of the newborn are colonized with *S. aureus*, although not frequently [5]. *S. aureus* can be seen mostly in the contact of colonized healthcare personnel with patients or in previously colonized patients. Mechanisms involved in the pathogenesis of these infections; adhesion of bacteria to the host, passage through anatomical barriers, inactivation of phagocytic cells, suppression of the humoral immune system of the relevant host and secretion of toxins. Factors affecting the formation of infection include the state of the host immune system, the number and virulence of microorganisms, and deterioration of skin and mucosal integrity [6]. In particular, patients using invasive medical devices and those with weakened immune systems are vulnerable to *S. aureus* infections [1]. Bonnal et al. reported that *S. aureus* is the causative agent in 18% of nosocomial bloodstream infections. Catheter-related bloodstream infection was detected in 38.2% of these cases [7]. It has been reported that healthcare-associated bloodstream infections caused by *S. aureus* can be used as a marker for general hand hygiene practices and compliance with infection control measures in hospitals [8].

2.2 *S. aureus* carriage

Nasal *S. aureus* carrier is an important source of infection for *S. aureus*, which can be transmitted by contact and airway. Conditions in which skin integrity is impaired such as burns and trauma may be predisposing factors, as well as foreign bodies such as prostheses and catheters are important risk factors. Contagion is also seen with the use of common items such as towels. Contamination is especially high in indoor areas. The reason for the higher rates of carriage in children and young people is stated to be more contact with respiratory secretions in these age groups. There is a strong relationship between nose and hand carriage in *S. aureus* infections.

In a study, when cultures were taken from the nose, perineum, groin, and armpit were compared, *S. aureus* growth was most common in the nose [9]. Although it increases during menstruation, it has been reported that 10% of women of childbearing age have *S. aureus* carriage in the vagina. It has been stated that while there may be different *S. aureus* strains in the same person, 69% of MRSA-positive patients may have colonization in more than one region [10]. *S. aureus* carriers are divided into four persistent, intermittent, transient carriers and non-carriers. While 10–35% of healthy individuals are persistent carriers and 20–75% are intermittent carriers, persistent carriers have a higher risk of developing infection due to the higher bacterial load. Intermittent carriers usually consist of healthcare workers, such as intensive care workers, who become decolonized between two shifts [11]. Persistent carriage is higher in children, and it turns into intermittent carriage between the ages of 10–20 [12]. Carriage is significantly higher in the presence of diabetes mellitus, hemodialysis or peritoneal dialysis patients, intravenous drug users, healthcare workers, inpatients, patients with eczematous skin disease, liver failure, and HIV infection [13].

Nosocomial infections are a global problem of patient loss. While nosocomial infections can occur in 5–10% of hospitalized patients in developed countries, this rate is around 25% in underdeveloped countries [14]. While the cases with *S. aureus* growth in blood culture were 5.5% of all cases, it was determined that 69% of the cases with only *S. aureus* growth consisted of samples obtained from intensive care units [15].

2.3 *S. aureus* resistance

While epidemics can be treated easily, some invasive infections such as bacteremia, septic arthritis, toxic shock syndrome, osteomyelitis and endocarditis may trigger, and these conditions may require inpatient treatment due to difficult complications. Antibiotic treatment is recommended against infections caused by pathogen in the body [16]. Clinically, treatment options are limited as *S. aureus* has acquired significant resistance to multiple classes of antibiotics [17]. It has shown significant potential in rapidly responding to the challenge posed by new antibiotics through the evolution of novel antimicrobial resistance mechanisms. The development of resistance in these pathogens occurs with enzymatic inactivation of the antimicrobial agent, change in the target site of the drug, efflux pump and sequestration of the antimicrobial agent [18].

S. aureus has developed resistance to almost all antibiotics that have been in clinical use for centuries as an important health problem for humanity. Antibiotic resistance of *S. aureus*, which started with sulfonamides, extended to glycopeptides. Resistance to penicillins, which came into use in the early 1940s, increased to 50% within five years with the selective selection of penicillinase-producing bacteria, and today it is 95% [19].

Methicillin resistance started to be seen in 1961, two years after it started to be used clinically. Later, resistance development was observed against clindamycin, chloramphenicol, tetracyclines, macrolides, rifampin, aminoglycosides and trimethoprim-sulfomethoxazole antibiotics, which were widely used in the 1970s. Quinolone resistance was detected in the 1980s [6]. Some studies have stated that horizontal gene transfer has a role in the rapid acquisition and spread of antibiotic resistance markers in *S. aureus* [2, 20]. Most of the clinical isolates of *S. aureus* have a plasmid ranging from 1 to 60 kb. These plasmids carry a variable number of resistance genes. Resistance to erythromycin, tetracycline and chloramphenicol is carried by small plasmids, while the larger ones carry multidrug resistance genes against α-lactam, macrolides and aminoglycosides [20]. The development of resistance to β-lactams (penicillin, oxacillin, methicillin and cephalosporin) in *S. aureus* occurs by the acquisition of a genomic island called the staphylococcal cassette chromosome (SCC*mec*) carrying *mecA* [21]. It has been determined that *S. aureus* penicillin resistance develops with the use of penicillin in treatment.

Penicillin resistance is mediated by the *blaZ* gene encoding β-lactamase enzymes [22]. Although penicillinase-resistant antibiotics such as methicillin have been used to overcome penicillin resistance, resistance to methicillin has emerged in *S. aureus* strains. It has been reported that β-lactam antibiotics cannot be used in the treatment of *Staphylococcus* infections due to methicillin resistance. Vancomycin, which is in the glycopeptide group, has been used in MRSA infections. In 2002, vancomycin resistance was also observed in *S. aureus* strains. This has made the treatment of *Staphylococcus* infections difficult [23].

2.4 Diseases caused by *S. aureus*

Bacteremias caused by staphylococci are examined in two groups hospital and community origin. While bacteremias that start 48–72 hours after hospitalization or within the first 10 days after hospital discharge are hospital-acquired, bacteremias that exist during hospitalization or develop within the first 24–72 hours are community-acquired. *S. aureus* bacteremia is seen at increasing rates in patients with staphylococcal diseases such as osteomyelitis and endocarditis, and in those using established medical devices. Prolonged hospital stays increase bacteremia due to *S. aureus* [6]. *S. aureus* causes common infections such as endocarditis, meningitis, impetigo, folliculitis, carbuncle, furuncle, cellulitis, bacteremia, pericarditis, pneumonia, osteomyelitis and septic arthritis. It also causes toxigenic syndromes such as toxic shock syndrome, septic shock, scalded skin syndrome, food poisoning [24]. It causes furuncle disease in areas where hair follicles are common, such as the face, neck, hips, and armpits [25]. *S. aureus* is one of the major causes of surgical wound infections. It occurs with the development of edema, erythema and pain around the wound after surgical intervention. In cases where there is no spread to deep tissues, removal of sutures, repetitive dressing and antibiotic treatment are sufficient [6, 10]. Scalded skin syndrome caused by exfoliative toxins produced by *S. aureus* strains and necrotizing pneumonia caused by Panton-Valentine leucocidin toxins can be life-threatening [26].

3. Methicillin-resistant *Staphylococcus aureus* (MRSA)

Resistance to antibiotics that are not hydrolyzed by β-lactamase is called methicillin resistance. *S. aureus* pathogens have gained methicillin resistance by horizontal transfer of *mecA*, which has low affinity for β-lactam antibiotics and encodes a modified penicillin-binding protein [27]. In MRSA, the acquisition of resistance occurs by mutation of the target gene in the chromosomes, efflux pump system, horizontal transfer of mobile genetic elements (MGEs), or enzymatic action of drugs, as in the case of penicillin [28]. PCR-based methods generally show the best sensitivity, although they have a higher cost and some risk of false-positive results.

3.1 Epidemiology

With the first use of penicillin in the treatment of staphylococcal infections in 1940, the morbidity and mortality of staphylococcal infections were significantly reduced. However, penicillin-resistant staphylococcal strains were reported for the first time in England in 1944, and many antibiotic resistances were described in staphylococci in the following years.

Staphylococci gain resistance by inhibiting β-lactam antibiotics by hydrolyzing the amide bond of the β-lactam ring with the enzyme β-lactamase (penicillinase) they produce. Methicillin, which is a penicillin derivative and resistant to β-lactamase enzyme, was removed from clinical use due to its serious side effects of causing interstitial nephritis, although it was the first antibiotic produced in 1959 and used in the clinic among β-lactamase antibiotics (methicillin, oxacillin, nafcillin, cloxacillin, dicloxacillin) [29]. MRSA spread rapidly in the 1960s and increased in many parts of the world.

The molecular epidemiology of *S. aureus* is largely determined by the succession of regionally dominant strains. Penicillin-resistant phage type 80 or 81 of *S. aureus* increased from 1953 to 1963 [30]. MRSA was identified in 1961, shortly after the introduction of methicillin, and MRSA outbreaks were reported at the same time [31]. Later, towards the end of the 1970s, MRSA infections began to be seen as endemic in Europe and America.

The prevalence of MRSA in the community is increasing due to the epidemic of community-associated MRSA strains. MRSA strains are divided into two groups community-acquired and hospital-acquired. Community-acquired MRSA cases can be seen in people who have not been treated in hospitals, young people, people in crowded communities, athletes and gyms. Community-acquired infections of MRSA usually occur in the form of skin and soft tissue infections.

There are 5 penicillin-binding proteins (PBPs) in methicillin-sensitive *S. aureus* (MSSA) bacteria. There are 7 MRSAs. PBP2a with a weight of 78 kDa is formed by the change of penicillin-binding protein. A gene known as *mec*A codes for this change [32]. The staphylococcal Cassette Chromosome (SCC) consists of the *mec* and *ccr* gene complexes located near the replication site. Methicillin resistance is caused by the *mec* gene complex [33]. MRSA is formed by the acquisition of a genomic island carrying the methicillin resistance determinant *mecA*. Since its discovery in the UK in the early 1960s, MRSA has been recognized worldwide as the most common cause of human, community and animal-associated infections. Significantly, too many antibiotics with MRSA resulted in a reduction of their therapeutic value, prolonging hospital stays [34].

3.2 MRSA carriage

The spread of MRSA infection usually occurs in the hospital setting. MRSA infection is carried into the hospital setting by patients or healthcare professionals. When MRSA infection is detected, risk factors such as hospitalization, close contact with a hospitalized person, and a history of chronic disease should be present [23]. MRSA colonization has been detected in nostrils, axillary, rectal, perirectal, oropharyngeal and intestinal samples [35]. Major identified risk factors for MRSA infections include surgery, dialysis, hospitalization, indwelling percutaneous devices such as central venous catheters or feeding tubes, or the patient's previous culture-proven MRSA infection. Healthcare-associated MRSA infection was defined as MRSA infection that developed 48 hours after hospitalization. MRSA is an important factor in healthcare-associated infections, especially in hospitalized patients.

Nasal carriage is important in the epidemiology of MRSA. Studies have indicated that the most suitable area where *S. aureus* bacteria is isolated is the nose. It has been stated that the bacteria are eradicated from other parts of the body in nasal treatment [36]. Almost any material that comes into contact with the skin, such as pens, mobile phones, white coats, and ties, can act as fomite in MRSA transmission. Colonization can continue for a long time. MRSA can also persist in the home setting and complicate eradication attempts [37]. Colonization is not stable as strains have been found to evolve and even migrate within the same host [38]. Nearly 80% of MRSA infections accumulate in the skin and soft tissues and spread rapidly. It has been shown that it causes diseases such as bursitis, osteomyelitis, arthritis, sinusitis, and urinary tract infection due to MRSA infection [39].

Individuals with MRSA colonization or carriers are at risk of developing an infection, and carriers are a source of person-to-person transmission. There are people prone to infection in healthcare facilities. Especially hospitals are areas where the use of antibiotics is high and places where there is frequent contact between people. These conditions facilitate the epidemic spread of MRSA in hospitals.

MRSA is still endemic in many healthcare facilities around the world and has become the focus of global infection control committees. When *S. aureus* strains isolated from hospitalized patients and wound samples were examined in the study, 75% of wound-borne strains, 51% of skin-borne strains and 74% of strains obtained from hospital beds were identified as MRSA. Yüksekkaya et al. stated that 48% of the cases with MRSA in blood culture were isolated from intensive care units, 47% from internal clinics, and 5% from surgical clinics [40]. In the study conducted by Zencir et al. on hospitalized patients, it was reported that 84.6% of the patients with MRSA growth in their blood culture were obtained from the intensive care units and 14.4% from the samples from other clinics [39].

Situations in which MRSA carriage increases include previously acquired MRSA carrier, being an intensive care unit worker, contact with a person carrying MRSA, taking care of a relative in need of home care, acne, chronic inflammatory bowel disease, contact with pets and raw meat [11]. Because MRSA is both commensal and pathogenic, attempting to eliminate the carrier following detection of MRSA colonization is predictive of the risk of subsequent infection [41].

3.3 Antibiotic resistance of MRSA

Methicillin resistance is due to the *mecA* gene. *mecA* is a gene encoding a novel penicillin-binding protein that confers resistance to all β-lactam antibiotics, including anti-staphylococcal penicillins, cephalosporins and carbapenems [42]. The emergence of multiple antibiotic resistance in MRSA infections prolongs the treatment period. MRSA infection usually spreads from the hospital [18]. Nosocomial infection is one of the most important factors in the multi-antibiotic resistance of MRSA. Detection of this agent will be an important step in infection control.

Glycopeptide antibiotics are generally preferred in the treatment of MRSA. The commonly preferred vancomycin. Daptomycin, quinopristin-dalfobristin, linezolid, tigecycline are other antibiotics used in the treatment. In a study by Kao et al. it was stated that 98.8% of 470 MRSA bacteria obtained from blood cultures were susceptible to daptomycin [43]. In a study conducted in the USA, it was reported that *S. aureus* bacteria were sensitive to daptomycin at a rate of 99.94% and 53.3% of these were MRSA [44]. In another study, the MRSA strains used were found to be sensitive to linezolid [45]. In a study on 67 MRSA strains, the antibiotics daptomycin, linezolid, teicoplanin, and vancomycin were used. It has been reported that daptomycin has 8 times more effective than vancomycin, 16 times more effect than teicoplanin and 4 times more effect than linezolid [46].

Patients with MRSA infection have higher mortality, longer hospital stays and higher healthcare costs, severe acute renal failure, hemodynamic instability, and long-term ventilator dependence than patients with methicillin-susceptible *Staphylococcus aureus* (MSSA) infection. While there are five penicillin-binding proteins in MSSA strains, a different PBP with a weight of 78 kDa, called PBP2a or PBP2', is additionally synthesized in resistant strains. This protein of different nature exhibits a low affinity for β-lactam antibiotics.

3.3.1 Chromosomal (intrinsic) methicillin resistance

Chromosomal mutations or deletions in the *mecA* gene system due to frequent or incorrect use of antibiotics may cause the suppressive function to be abolished in *S. aureus* strains and cause continuous production of PBP2a [47].

Chromosomal methicillin resistance occurs in three ways. These;

1. Homogeneous resistance is when each bacterium in the colony has the *mecA* gene, can synthesize PBP2a, and shows a high degree of methicillin resistance.

2. Heterogeneous resistance is the condition in which high methicillin resistance is found in only one of 106 to 108 bacteria, although all bacteria in the colony carry the *mecA* gene. It is common in the clinic. The fact that PBP2a expression is not strongly induced in strains carrying normal regulatory genes (*mecA, mecR1* and *mecl*) and its induction is much slower causes some strains to be methicillin-sensitive despite carrying the *mecA* gene. The high methicillin resistance seen in this type of resistance is in a region outside the *mec* gene; It is the result of an additional chromosomal mutation defined as *chr*, which is thought to be located at the *hmr* locus.

3. Eagle-tip resistance, strains susceptible to methicillin at low methicillin concentrations become resistant to methicillin at high concentrations. This is presumed to be the result of intact *mecA* regulator genes inducing PBP2a synthesis at high methicillin concentrations [29].

The high prevalence of MRSA is attributed to its toxin production, rapid spread, and capacity to have multiple antibiotic resistance markers. This causes an increasing burden on limited health service. The rapid spread of natural resistance genes among pathogenic strains reduces the clinical importance of many drugs in a short time.

3.4 Treatment

MRSA causes a challenging, versatile and unpredictable infection. Genetic adaptation capacity and the rapid emergence of strong epidemic strains pose a great threat to health. Studies evaluating genomics, epigenetics, transcription, proteomics, and metabolomics in animal models and patients with a variety of MRSA are crucial to the understanding and treatment of MRSA infection [41]. The hands of hospital staff are important in the spread of MRSA. Recently, methicillin resistance has increased worldwide. The fight against MRSA in the hospital setting is a crucial step in starting the treatment process right away. Immediate initiation of MRSA treatment with early detection will reduce the incidence. In addition to appropriate antimicrobial therapy, infectious disease consultation will reduce mortality from MRSA bacteremia.

An important pathogen in nosocomial infections, MRSA has also gained importance as a community source. The risk of colonization and infection is higher in patients using antibiotics. MRSA is methicillin-resistant and resistant to all β-lactam antibiotics. It is mentioned that there is resistance to clindamycin, macrolides, tetracycline, chloramphenicol and aminoglycosides. Mortality rate in MRSA infections is much higher than in MSSA. Patients infected with MRSA are hospitalized for more time in intensive care treatment. Multiple antibiotics effective against MRSA have been approved by the FDA since 2014. However, the sustained and high mortality rate from invasive MRSA infection suggests the need for high-quality studies to determine the optimal management for these patients. In order to carry out such studies, it is necessary to establish a clinical research network. By expanding the research area, the clinical impact of this pathogen can be reduced.

4. Conclusion

Hospital infections not only affect the patient but also negatively affect the companions and healthcare workers. Many problems such as an increase in morbidity and mortality, decrease in quality of life, loss in cost and productivity, and prolongation of hospital stay are caused by nosocomial infections. The major challenge in the treatment of *S. aureus* infection is the lack of suitable therapeutic agents, as pathogens develop resistance to almost all antibiotics. The increasing problem of antibiotic resistance in hospital infections caused by MRSA has become an important health problem that increases its severity worldwide. As a result, there is an increase in the rates of healthcare-associated infections caused by *S. aureus* and MRSA. This increase can be prevented by providing adequate training on hygiene, increasing compliance with standard infection control measures, and improving the rational use of antibiotics.

Author details

Songul Cetik Yildiz
Department of Medical Services and Techniques, Mardin Artuklu University, Vocational Higher School of Health Services, Mardin, Turkey

*Address all correspondence to: songulcetik@gmail.com

References

[1] Lee AS, De Lencastre H, Garau J, Kluytmans J, Malhotra-Kumar S, Peschel A, et al. Methicillin-resistant *Staphylococcus aureus*. Nature Reviews. Disease Primers. 2018;**4**(1):1-23

[2] Bitrus AA, Zunita Z, Bejo SK, Othman S, Nadzir NA. In vitro transfer of methicillin resistance determinants mec A from methicillin resistant *Staphylococcus aureus* (MRSA) to methicillin susceptible *Staphylococcus aureus* (MSSA). BMC Microbiology. 2017;**17**(1):83

[3] Yuksekdag Z, Baltacı N. *Staphylococcus aureus* Türlerinde Biyofilm ve Biyofilm Oluşumundan Sorumlu Genler. Turk Mikrobiyol Cemiy Derg. 2013;**43**(3):77-83

[4] Shaw L, Golonka E, Potempa J, Foster SJ. The role and regulation of the extracellular proteases of *Staphylococcus aureus*. Microbiologica. 2004;**150**(1):217-228

[5] Gungor S, Uzun B, Yurtsever S, Baran N. Kan Kültürlerinde İzole Edilen *Staphylococcus aureus* suşlarında antibiyotiklere direnç. ANKEM Derg. 2012;**26**(4):171-175

[6] Tunger A. *Staphylococcus aureus*: Mikrobiyoloji, patogenez ve epidemiyoloji. In: Ulusoy S, Usluer G, Ünal S, editors. Gram-pozitif bakteri infeksiyonları. Ankara: Bilimsel Tıp Yayınevi; 2004. pp. 9-68

[7] Bonnal C, Birgand G, Lolom I, Diamantis S, Dumortier C, L'Heriteau F, et al. *Staphylococcus aureus* healthcare associated bacteraemia: An indicator of catheter related infections. Médecine et Maladies Infectieuses. 2015;**45**:84-88

[8] Kılıç KE, Demircan ŞA, Kinikli S, Cesur S, Büyükdemirci A, Hatipoğlu AC, et al. Sağlık bakımı ilişkili enfeksiyonlarda *Staphylococcus aureus* dağılımının irdelenmesi: 6 yıllık deneyim. Journal of Medical Palliative Care. 2022;**3**(1):39-43

[9] Zimakoff J, Pedersen FB, Bergen L, Baago-Nielsen J, Daldorph B, Espersen F, et al. *Staphylococcus aureus* carriage and infections among patients in four haemo- and peritoneal-dialysis centres in Denmark. The Danish Study Group of Peritonitis in Dialysis. The Journal of Hospital Infection. 1996;**33**(4):289-300

[10] Dundar V, Dundar DO. Stafilokok Enfeksiyonları. Enfeksiyon Hastalıkları ve Mikrobiyolojisi. İstanbul: Nobel Tıp Kitapevleri; 2008:2065-2077

[11] Dulon M, Peters C, Schablon A, Nienhaus A. MRSA carriage among healthcare workers in non-outbreak settings in Europe and the United States: A systematic review. BMC Infectious Diseases. 2014;**3**(14):363

[12] Saxena S, Singh K, Talwar V. Methicillin-resistant *Staphylococcus aureus* prevalance in community in the East Delhi area. Japanese Journal of Infectious Diseases. 2003;**56**:54-56

[13] Murray PR, Rosenthal KS, Pfaller PA. Medical Microbiology. 4th ed. Philadelphia: Elsevier; 2005. pp. 203-236

[14] Fridkin SK, Welbel SF, Weisten RA. Magnitude and prevention of nosocomial infection in Intensive Care Unit. Infectious Disease Clinics of North America. 1997;**11**:479-496

[15] Ozkaya E, Tumer S, Kirisci O, Caliskan A, Erdogmus P. Son iki yılda

Kahramanmaraş Necip Fazıl Şehir Hastanesi'nde kan kültürlerinden izole edilen mikroorganizmalar ve antibiyotik duyarlılıklarının değerlendirilmesi. Türk Hijiyen ve Deneysel Biyoloji Dergisi. 2015;**72**:115-122

[16] Cadena J, Frei CR, Thinwa J, Walter EA. Risk factors for the development of active methicillin-resistant *Staphylococcus aureus* (MRSA) infection in patients colonized with MRSA at hospital admission. American Journal of Infection Control. 2016;**44**:1617-1621

[17] Lakhundi S, Zhang K. Methicillin-resistant *Staphylococcus aureus*: Molecular characterization, evolution, and epidemiology. Clinical Microbiology Reviews. 2018;**31**(4):e00020-e00018

[18] Bitrus AA, Peter OM, Abbas MA, Goni MD. *Staphylococcus aureus*: A review of antimicrobial resistance mechanisms. Veterinary Sciences. 2018;**4**(2):43-54

[19] Dundar V. Metisiline dirençli stafilokok infeksiyonları. Klin Derg. 2000;**13**:26-27

[20] Sabet NS, Subramaniam G, Navaratnam P, Sekaran SD. In vitro mecA gene transfer among *Staphylococcus aureus* in Malaysian clinical isolates. African Journal of Biotechnology. 2014;**11**:385-390

[21] Bitrus AA, Zunita Z, Khairani-Bejo S, Othman S, Ahmad Nadzir NA. Staphylococcal cassette chromosome *mec* (SCC*mec*) and characterization of the attachment site (attB) of methicillin resistant *Staphylococcus aureus* (MRSA) and methicillin susceptible *Staphylococcus aureus* (MSSA) isolates. Microbial Pathogenesis. 2018b;**123**:323-329

[22] Page MGP. Beta-lactam Antibiotics. Antibiotic Discovery and Development. vol. 9781461414. US: Springer; 2012. pp. 79-117

[23] Weems JJ. The many faces of *Staphylococcus aureus* infection: Recognizing and managing its life-threatening manifestations. Postgraduate Medicine. 2001;**110**(4):24-36

[24] Tong SYC, Davis JS, Eichenberger E, Holland TL, Fowler VG. *Staphylococcus aureus* infections: Epidemiology, pathophysiology, clinical manifestations, and management. Clinical Microbiology Reviews. 2015;**28**(3):603-661

[25] Winn W, Allen S, Janda W, Koneman E, Procop G, Schreckenberger P, et al. Gram-Positive Coccipart I. In: Winn WC, editor. Konemans Color Atlas and Textbook of Diagnostic Microbiology. Baltimore: Lippincott Williams & Wilkins; 2006. pp. 623-671

[26] Labandeira-Rey M, Couzon F, Boisset S, Brown EL, Bes M, Benito Y, et al. *Staphylococcus aureus* Panton-Valentine leucocidin causes necrotizing pneumonia. Science. 2007;**315**:1130-1133

[27] Stojanov M, Sakwinska O, Moreillon P. Expression of SCC*mec* cassette chromosome recombinases in methicillin-resistant *Staphylococcus aureus* and *Staphylococcus epidermidis*. The Journal of Antimicrobial Chemotherapy. 2013;**68**(4):749-757

[28] Alekshun MN, Levy SB. Molecular mechanisms of antibacterial multidrug resistance. Cell. 2007;**128**(6):1037-1050

[29] Unal S. *Staphylococcus aureus*: Direnç Mekanizmaları. In: Ulusoy S, Usluer G, Ünal S, editors. Gram-pozitif bakteri infeksiyonları. Ankara: Bilimsel Tıp Yayinevi; 2004. pp. 23-38

[30] DeLeo FR, Adam DK, Chen L, Wardenburg JB, Kobayashi SD,

Mathema B, et al. Molecular differentiation of historic phage- type 80/81 and contemporary epidemic *Staphylococcus aureus*. Proceedings of the National Academy Science USA. 2011;**108**:18091-18096

[31] Benner EJ, Kayser F. Growing clinical significance of methicillin-resistant *Staphylococcus aureus*. Lancet. 1968;**292**(7571):741-744

[32] Deurenberg RH, Vink C, Kalenic S, Friedrich AW, Bruggeman CA, Stobberingh EE. The molecular evolution of methicillin-resistant *Staphylococcus aureus*. Clinical Microbiology and Infection. 2007;**13**(3):222-235

[33] Hanssen AM, Ericson Sollid JU. SCC*mec* in staphylococci: Genes on the move. FEMS Immunology Medicine Microbiology. 2006;**46**(1):8-20

[34] Purrello SM, Daum RS, Edwards GF, Lina G, Lindsay J, Peters G, et al. Meticillin-resistant *Staphylococcus aureus* (MRSA) update: New insights into bacterial adaptation and therapeutic targets. Journal of Global Antimicrobial Resistance. 2014;**2**(2):61-69

[35] Gagnaire J, Verhoeven PO, Grattard F, Rigaill J, Lucht F, Pozzetto B, et al. Epidemiology and clinical relevance of *Staphylococcus aureus* intestinal carriage: A systematic review and meta-analysis. Expert Review of Anti-Infective Therapy. 2017;**15**:767-785

[36] Parras F, Guerrero MC, Bouza E, Blazquez MJ, Moreno S, Menarguez MC, et al. Comparative study of mupirocin and oral cotrimoxazole plus topical fusidic acid in eradication of nasal carriage of methicillin resistant *Staphylococcus aureus*. Antimicrobial Agents and Chemotherapy. 1995;**39**:175-179

[37] Eells SJ, David MZ, Taylor A, Ortiz N, Kumar N, Sieth J, et al. Persistent environmental contamination with USA300 methicillin resistant *Staphylococcus aureus* and other pathogenic strain types in households with *S. aureus* skin infections. Infection Control and Hospital Epidemiology. 2014;**35**:1373-1382

[38] Azarian T, Daum RS, Petty LA, Steinbeck JL, Yin Z, Nolan D, et al. Intrahost evolution of methicillinresistant *Staphylococcus aureus* USA300 among individuals with reoccurring skin and soft- tissue infections. The Journal of Infectious Diseases. 2016;**214**:895-905

[39] Zenci M, Arı A, Yılmaz N, Avcı M, Çalık Ş, Coşkuner SA, et al. Antibiotic susceptibility of methicillin resistant *Staphylococcus aureus* strains, clinical features of patients and factors affecting mortality. Ankem Derg. 2016;**30**:18-23

[40] Yuksekkaya S, Opus A, Guvenc HI, Kaya M, Akkaya O, Guzelant A, et al. Evaluation of antimicrobial susceptibility of *Staphylococcus aureus* strains isolated from blood cultures in Konya Training and Research Hospital between the years 2009-2013. Ankem Derg. 2017;**31**:1-6

[41] Turner NA, Sharma-Kuinkel BK, Maskarinec SA, Eichenberger EM, Shah PP, Carugati M, et al. Methicillin-resistant *Staphylococcus aureus*: An overview of basic and clinical research. Nature Reviews. Microbiology. 2019;**17**(4):203-218

[42] Monaco M, de Araujo FP, Cruciani M, Coccia EM, Pantosti A. Worldwide Epidemiology and Antibiotic Resistance of *Staphylococcus aureus*, *Staphylococcus aureus* Microbiology, Pathology, Immunology, Therapy and Prophylaxis. Switzerland: Springer International Publishing AG; 2016. pp. 21-56

[43] Kao TM, Wang JT, Weng CM, Chen YC, Chang SC. In vitro activity of linezolid, tigecycline, and daptomycin on methicillin-resistant *Staphylococcus aureus* blood isolates from adult patients, 2006-2008: Stratified analysis by vancomycin mic. Journal of Microbiology, Immunology, and Infection. 2011;**44**(5):346-351

[44] Sader HS, Moet GJ, Farrell DJ, Jones RN. Antimicrobial susceptibility of daptomycin and comparator agents tested against methicillin-resistant *Staphylococcus aureus* and vancomycin-resistant enterococci: Trend analysis of A 6-year period in US Medical Centers (2005-2010). Diagnostic Microbiology and Infectious Disease. 2011;**70**(3):412-416

[45] Pelitli TS, Cesur S, Kinikli S, Irmak H, Demiroz AP, Karakoc E. Evaluation of vancomycin, teicoplanin, linezolide and tigecycline susceptibilities of nosocomicol methicillin-resistant *Staphylococcus* strains by e-test. Mikrobiyoloji Bülteni. 2011;**45**(4):758-761

[46] Diler GO. Daptomisinin metisiline dirençli *Staphylococcus aureus* İzolatlarında invitro etkinliğinin araştırılması. Bolu: Abant Izzet Baysal Üniversitesi; 2016

[47] Gür D. Bakterilerde antibiyotiklere karşı direnç. In: Topçu AW, Söyletir G, Doğanay M, editors. Enfeksiyon hastalıkları ve mikrobiyolojisi. İstanbul: Nobel Tıp Kitabevleri; 2008. pp. 243-257

Chapter 2

Multidrug-Resistant *Staphylococcus aureus* as Coloniser in Healthy Individuals

Asdren Zajmi, Fathimath Shiranee, Shirley Gee Hoon Tang, Mohammed A.M. Alhoot and Sairah Abdul Karim

Abstract

Staphylococcus aureus is a common human pathogen that can cause mild superficial infections to deep-seated abscesses and sepsis. One of the characteristics of *S. aureus* is the ability to colonise healthy individuals while leaving them asymptomatic. These carriers' risk harbouring an antibiotic-resistant strain that may be harmful to the individual and the community. *S. aureus* carriage in healthcare personnel is being studied extensively in many parts of the world. However, the relationship between colonisation and disease among those with no previous exposure to healthcare remains untouched. Colonisation of the nasal cavity and its surrounding by pathogenic organisms such as *S. aureus* leads to the increased risk of infection. Hospital-acquired infections associated with *S. aureus* infections are common and studies related to these types of infections among various study groups are largely documented. However, over the last decade, an increase in community-associated methicillin-resistant *S. aureus* has been noted, increasing the need to identify the prevalence of the organism among healthy individuals and assessing the antibiotic resistance patterns. Systemic surveillance of the community for colonisation of *S. aureus* and identifying the antibiotic-resistant pattern is critical to determine the appropriate empiric antibiotic treatment.

Keywords: *Staphylococcus aureus*, multidrug resistance *S. aureus*, community acquired-MRSA, healthy individuals, antibiotic resistance

1. Introduction

S. aureus is the most significant pathogen within the genus *Staphylococcus* and a major human pathogen capable of causing a wide variety of infections [1]. This pathogen was first discovered by a Scottish surgeon from a surgical abscess [2]. *S. aureus* is a Gram-positive, catalase and coagulase producing, oxidase negative, non-spore-forming cocci [3]. *S. aureus* can interact with its host as a commensal member of the microbiota [4] or act as an opportunistic pathogen leading to a wide range of community and hospital-associated infections [5–7]. The nose (anterior nares) is the most frequent ecological niche of *S. aureus* carriage, but this bacterium can also colonise multiple body sites including pharynx [8–10], skin, rectum, vagina, axilla, and gastrointestinal tract [11]. It was found that approximately 20–30% of the human population harboured this bacterium persistently and asymptomatically in the anterior nares [4].

Nasal colonisation of *S. aureus* has shown to be an increased risk factor for the development of community-acquired or nosocomial infections by two to tenfold [12]. Most community-acquired *S. aureus* infections happen due to autoinfection from anterior nares, skin or both [13]. Transmission of *S. aureus* may happen through contaminated objects and surfaces although the main route of transmission is mainly from a colonised or individual having an infection with *S. aureus* [14]. *S. aureus* is also known to cause mild superficial infections to deep-seated abscesses and life-threatening sepsis [11]. Additionally, it has been documented that persistent nasal colonisation by *S. aureus* increased the risk for subsequent infections and this situation became even more complicated in immunocompromised and hospitalised individuals which can lead to invasive infections with high morbidity and mortality rates [15, 16].

Antimicrobial resistance has caused a significant challenge to modern medicine as well as to the possibility of effective treatment of infectious diseases. The emergence of antibiotic resistance among *S. aureus* has been a problem since the identification of penicillinase-producing *S. aureus* just two years post-discovery of Penicillin [17]. Like other bacteria, *S. aureus* also develops resistance on exposure to antibiotics, leading to resistant strains [18]. The antibiotic resistance crisis has been accelerated by the misuse and overuse of antibiotics leading to a 'silent pandemics' [19]. It has been reported that infections caused by antibiotic-resistant strains of *S. aureus* have reached epidemic proportions worldwide. Several studies have found that the overall burden of staphylococcal disease in both hospital and community settings, especially that caused by methicillin-resistant *S. aureus* strains (MRSA), has increased in various countries including China, Brazil, India and Turkey as well as Malaysia [20–25]. Some previous studies have shown that the emergence of community-associated MRSA (CA-MRSA) strains was one of the major causes of skin and soft-tissue infections [26]. The rapid spread of CA-MRSA strains has been reported in some other countries with a historically low prevalence of MRSA such as Norway, Denmark, Asia, Canada, Australia, Sweden and Finland [27–29]. CA-MRSA strains have demonstrated a remarkable diversity in the number of different clones that have been characterised [14].

In Asia, the multidrug-resistant strains of *S. aureus* particularly MRSA have become endemic in most hospitals and poses a major threat to public health and treatment challenge to physicians due to its limited therapeutic options [30]. Multidrug-resistant *S. aureus* such as MRSA is no longer confined to patients with known risk factors or exposure to healthcare settings. Several reports about MRSA infection have increased the public concerns about the implications of the transmission of *S. aureus* among healthy individuals. It has been found that MRSA carriage in healthy individuals is a major asymptomatic reservoir that led to the wide spread of MRSA within the community [31–33]. In Malaysia, a recent study conducted by Suhaili, Azis [34] showed that a total of 49 of *S. aureus* strains isolated from 200 healthy undergraduate students in the year 2012 and 2013 yielded eight erythromycin-resistant isolates. Among these eight isolates, six were found to harbour the *msrA* gene and one isolate carried the *ermC* gene [34].

2. Colonisation

The colonisation of the human body with *S. aureus* is closely linked with serious blood infections to minor skin infections [35]. The anterior nares happen to be the most common site of *S. aureus* colonisation with the nasal cavity and vestibule harbouring *S. aureus* equally [36, 37]. The likelihood of *S. aureus* being transferred from the nasal site to other body parts via hand transfer is high [38]. Nasal carriage of *S. aureus* varying from 20% to >50% was detected in studies conducted in different parts of the world [39–43].

Various other sites colonisation the *S. aureus* has been documented including the oropharynx, skin, vagina, rectum, gastrointestinal tract and axilla [12]. In a study conducted among healthy individuals in the Iowa United States, nasal swabs and oropharyngeal swabs were collected, revealing a higher prevalence of *S. aureus* [44]. The authors of this study suggest that the addition of sites other than the anterior nares increases the chances of identifying prevalence rates and genotypic differences among *S. aureus* in different parts of the body [44]. A study conducted by Azmi, Adnan [45] to identify the prevalence of *S. aureus* in the oral cavity of healthy adults in Malaysia explained an increase in the occurrence of *S. aureus* with a significant association with the presence of dental prostheses. With every rise in colonisation, the risk of infection increases, indicating the importance of identifying the different areas and colonisation rates [45]. The colonisation of multiple anatomical sites can lead to horizontal gene transfer and antibiotic resistance between co-colonising strains [46].

S. aureus colonisation rates can vary among individuals with different clinical conditions and having an underlying condition can be a significant factor associated with nasal colonisation [12, 47]. Patients with diabetes mellitus (DM) show a high prevalence of MRSA nasal colonisation [12]. Supportive to this finding are studies conducted by Bhoi, Otta [48] and Lin, Lin [49], where DM patients had a higher rate of MRSA colonisation compared to healthy individuals. This type of colonisation can lead to more severe conditions such as foot ulcers in DM patients [49]. Lin and the team researched diabetic patients in Taiwan to assess the concordance between colonisation and MRSA colonisation, revealing nasal carriage of MRSA to be a significant risk factor for foot ulcers in DM patients [49]. A similar study in New York with patients undergoing total hip arthroplasty and knee arthroplasty showed a high carrier rate of *S. aureus* [50]. Hidron, Kempker [51] described that an individual's chance of colonisation with *S. aureus* is increased by 17% in HIV positive patients and 1.3% - 5.3% in patients admitted in hospital settings [51]. A higher prevalence of *S. aureus* colonisation (44.0%) was observed among HIV infected individuals in a case-control study done in India [52]. Apart from HIV patients affected with comorbidities such as obesity and diabetes can also have a higher *S. aureus* carrier rate [12]. A study conducted among the Norwegian population showed a vast increase in *S. aureus* colonisation with the increase in body mass index (BMI) (for each 2.5 kg/m^2 a 7% increase) [53]. However, the prevalence rate of *S. aureus* is not similar to all chronic diseases. *S. aureus* nasal colonisation rate had no significant difference among rheumatoid arthritis patients and the general population [54].

The prevalence rates of *S. aureus* in healthy individuals vary from population to population with certain risk factors making them more prone to colonisation [35]. Studies including healthy individuals from the general community or university/college campus in Iran, China, Saudi Arabia and Taiwan showed prevalence rates of 30.16%, 24.7%, 37.0% and 22.0% respectively [40, 41, 43, 55]. Findings from the refugee community indicated a higher prevalence rate of 44.0% in Nepal and 51.2% in Portugal, indicating the variance in prevalence among different populations and geographical distributions [42, 56]. Curry and his team observed that the prevalence of *S. aureus* colonisation can be increased with living in confined spaces with limited exposure to external environments. This study was conducted among Navy crew members in an assault ship during a 3-week training session. Among the 400 participants, 59.7% was colonised with *S. aureus* [57]. Prior exposure to antibiotics also poses a risk factor for *S. aureus* colonisation [58]. A case-control study conducted from 2005 to 2010 revealed that 37% of patients with MRSA infection were exposed to antibiotics three months before [59].

Research conducted among healthy individuals in Malaysia revealed a low prevalence rate of *S. aureus* from nasal swabs of medical students (9.24%) and dental students (18.0%) [60, 61]. A higher prevalence of *S. aureus* was observed from oral cavity samples (40.0%) and hand swab samples of food handlers (95.0%) from Ampang Jaya and Klang Valley respectively [45, 62].

3. A pathogen of concern

S. aureus is a fast-evolving Gram-positive coccus and one of the most typical opportunistic pathogens identified [63]. *S. aureus* has been a leading cause of nosocomial infection till the identification of epidemiologically distinct colonies in community settings [64]. *S. aureus* is responsible for hospital-acquired infections (HAI) such as surgical site infections, nosocomial pneumonia and central line-associated bloodstream infections (CLABSI) which can lead to life-threatening situations [65]. Several studies and texts describe *S. aureus* among most common isolates responsible for hospital-acquired infections [66–69]. With stringent measures, a reduction in HAI with *S. aureus* is seen but community-acquired infections are still on the rise [70, 71].

S. aureus is frequently isolated from skin and soft tissue infections (SSTIs). A study conducted in Greece from 2014 to 2018 identified the presence of *S. aureus* in 46.4% of patients with SSTIs [72]. *S. aureus* was isolated from 62% of all wound or abscess cultures received at a medical treatment facility in the U.S from 2005 to 2010 [73]. Kumar and their team also reported a high percentage of *S. aureus* (75.0%) isolated from wound abscess of adults and children aged 6 months to 84 years [74]. Apart from SSTIs *S. aureus* has also been isolated from patients with mastitis. Cultures performed on breast milk from patients with mastitis revealed the presence of *S. aureus* in 19.8% and 38.2% of the sample from studies conducted in China and Italy respectively [75, 76].

S. aureus infections become more serious when it enters the bloodstream, and this type of infection tends to be more fatal and is regarded as a significant cause of morbidity and mortality in infected patients [77]. Marra, Camargo [78] reported *S. aureus* as the primary organism responsible for nosocomial bloodstream infections (15.4%) in Brazil with a crude mortality rate of 31.0% [78]. Similar results were also seen in a study conducted with blood samples received from laboratories of 25 European countries where *S. aureus* was the pathogen in over 3000 samples [79]. Conditions associated with *S. aureus* bacteraemia such as infective endocarditis and osteomyelitis also remains as important metastatic infections as these can add to the morbidity and mortality rates. An observational study conducted at a Danish hospital included patients admitted with *S. aureus* bacteraemia (SAB) to determine the prevalence of

No.	Author, year	Purpose/Aims/Goals	Approach/Method/Experiment	Dataset/Sampling	Findings/Results
1	(Ahmadi et al., 2019)	Evaluate nasal colonisation of MRSA in healthy individuals	Cross-sectional study *S. aureus* isolated from nasal swabs identified by the gram and biochemical testing. ABST by agar disk diffusion PCR for *mec*A, SCC*mec*, *pvl* encoding genes	600 randomly chosen individuals based on non-probability haphazard sampling type	High incidence of CA-MRSA in asymptomatic individuals
2	(Abroo et al., 2017)	Investigate prevalence, antimicrobial susceptibility, and molecular characteristics of CA-MRSA	*S. aureus* cultures identified by gram film & biochemicals. PCR for species-specific genes ABST by disc diffusion	Nasal swabs of 700 healthy student volunteers	High frequency of *S. aureus* nasal carriers with multidrug resistance detected
3	(Hanif & Hassan, 2019)	Evaluation of sensitivity value of *S. aureus* against different antibiotics	*S. aureus* was identified using gram smear and biochemical testing. ABST by disc diffusion	265 clinical *S. aureus* isolates from different sources	An increase in an overall antibiotic-resistant trend seen
4	(Eibach et al., 2017)	Identify demographic and season-specific carriage rates, clonal types, virulence markers, and antibiotic susceptibilities of *S. aureus* isolates	*S. aureus* from nasal swabs identified by the gram and biochemical testing. ABST by disk diffusion Spa -typing for virulence testing and PCR for TSST, *mec*, *mec*C, *mec*A	544 children <15 years, nasal swab sample collected on admission	The nasal carriage was dependent on age and season. Multidrug resistance within *S. aureus* increased comparatively.
5	(Chen et al., 2016)	Investigate the nasal carriage, molecular characterisation, and antimicrobial resistance of *S. aureus* in newly admitted inpatients	*S. aureus* identified based on biochemical testing, molecular identification by identifying *nuc* gene, ABST by disk diffusion	Nasal swabs from 292 patients 48 hrs within the admission	Nasal colonisation of CA-MRSA and H.A.- MRSA detected with high resistance to erythromycin among *S. aureus* isolates
6	(Chen et al., 2017)	Determine prevalence and risk factors of *S. aureus* nasal carriage	Cross-sectional study Identification of *S. aureus* by biochemical testing and MRSA by cefoxitin and PCR for *mec*A, *pvl*, *sea*, and *seb* genes ABST by disk diffusion Questionnaire to identify risk	Two hundred ninety-five nasal swabs were taken from university teachers, undergraduates, middle school, salesclerks, and retirees.	Prevalence of *S. aureus* more likely in males aged 20–30 with irregular nasal cleaning behaviour. Molecular heterogeneity among *S. aureus* isolates seen

No.	Author, year	Purpose/Aims/Goals	Approach/Method/Experiment	Dataset/Sampling	Findings/Results
7	(Conceição et al., 2019)	Determine MRSA colonisation rates and significant risk factors for *S. aureus* carriage, also to characterise *S. aureus* clonal population, antibiotic resistance, and virulence	MRSA was confirmed by PCR amplification of *nuc, mec*A, and *spa* genes. ABST by disk diffusion method. Characterisation by PFGE, spa typing, MLST, SCCmec typing, and *pvl* detection	Nasal swabs from 84 individuals >18 years old meeting the eligibility criteria (living without facilities to cook and intact nasal mucosa)	*S. aureus* colonisation rate was high with low MRSA colonisation together with a pool of highly transmissible ST398-t1451 MSSA lineage
8	(Laub et al., 2018)	Estimate *S. aureus* nasal carriage rate in healthy children population and characterise strains by molecular techniques	*S. aureus* was identified by biochemical testing. PCR to detect *nuc*A and *mec*A gene. ABST performed by MIC method	Nasal swabs of 1390 healthy children (3 to 7) year old from 20 different day-care centres	A high carriage rate of *S. aureus* was seen in preschool children, but the CA-MRSA carriage rate was low. All MRSA isolates belonged to ST45
9	(Le et al., 2018)	Determine whether analysis of a single *S. aureus* from an individual is adequate to determine the carrier status of a particular strain or characteristics of *S. aureus*	Biochemical testing to identify *S. aureus. Spa*, *mec*A, and *scn* gene identified by PCR. ABST was done by disc diffusion method	19 participants (190 isolates total) were selected from a cohort of industrial hog operation workers and household members	Relying on testing one isolate may not capture the variable characteristics of *S. aureus*
10	(Ronga et al., 2019)	Evaluate cumulative antibiograms of *S. aureus* clinical isolates	Biochemical identification and antibiotic susceptibility by VITEK MSTM and VITEK 2 System TM	1229 samples from hospitalised and ambulatory care patients	Higher resistance rates were detected for penicillin, oxacillin, levofloxacin, erythromycin, and clindamycin. The difference in annual resistance was not statistically significant
11	(Okamo et al., 2016)	Determine the prevalence and antimicrobial susceptibility profile of S. aureus and MRSA and identify the association of *S. aureus* nasal carriage with demographic and clinical characteristics	Cross-sectional study. Questionnaire to collect demographic and clinical information. S. aureus identification by gram and biochemical testing. ABST by disk diffusion	Nasal swabs of 314 medical students were randomly selected. Pre-clinical (n = 166) and clinical (n = 148)	High prevalence of *S. aureus* carriage among medical students with a low prevalence of MRSA

No.	Author, year	Purpose/Aims/Goals	Approach/Method/Experiment	Dataset/Sampling	Findings/Results
12	(Ansari et al., 2016)	Assess the nasal carriage rate of *S. aureus*, MRSA and identify antimicrobial susceptibility and associated risk factors	Cross-sectional study. *S. aureus* was identified by biochemical methods and ABST done using disk diffusion.	The nasal swab of 200 medical students who were not exposed to a clinical setting	No significant association with *S. aureus* carriage and socio-demographic and habitual risk factors. URTIs can increase the carriage of *S. aureus* and MRSA
13	(Gong et al., 2017)	Describe the prevalence of S. *aureus*, its antibiotic resistance, and the presence of *mec*A and PVL genes	*S. aureus* was identified by biochemical test and latex agglutination. ABST testing by disk diffusion and strain testing for *mec*A by PCR	Nasal swabs of 314 healthy Tibetan children living at an altitude of 2500–4100 meters.	Prevalence of *S. aureus* increasing among the population with detection of methicillin-resistant strains
14	(Wang et al., 2017)	Elucidate the carriage rate of *S. aureus* and MRSA among competitive sports participants	*S. aureus* was identified, and ABST was done with disk diffusion. Molecular characterisation was done by PFGE and MLST. A questionnaire was34filled for demographics and risk factors	The nasal swabs of 259 students; 120 non-athletes, and 139 athletes	No significant difference in the nasal carriage of MRSA among athletes and non-athletes. The carriage rate of *S. aureus* among non-athletes and athletes was the same.
15	(Suhaili et al., 2018)	Assess antimicrobial susceptibility profiles of S. aureus isolated from a healthy population and determine the prevalence of constitutive and inducible clindamycin resistance	*S. aureus* confirmed with gram and biochemical testing. ABST by disk diffusion and molecular detection of virulence genes and antimicrobial resistance genes by PCR	Nasal swabs of 200 university students in health sciences	The presence of *pvl*-positive MSSA carriage and MLSB suggest the importance of nasal carriage as a transmission of disease.
16	(Azis et al., 2017)	Assess and compare the antimicrobial susceptibility pattern of *S. aureus*, also to identify the molecular and methicillin resistance-associated genotypes of *S. aureus*.	*S. aureus was* identified by the gram and biochemical testing, ABST by disc diffusion, and E-test. *mec*A, SCCmec, *spa* gene identification by PCR	120 university students, nasal swabs collected, and persistent carriers identified (n = 39)	Persistent antimicrobial patterns and limited methicillin resistance-associate genotypes were observed.
17	(Lim Fong et al., 2018)	Prevalence and antibiotic sensitivity profile of *S. aureus* and MRSA isolates from medical students	Culture and biochemical testing for the identification of *S. aureus.* Disk diffusion and Brilliance MRSA agar for ABST	60 medical students, 24 preclinical and 36 clinical, nasal swabs collected	High prevalence of *S. aureus* among medical students and low prevalence of MRSA

No.	Author, year	Purpose/Aims/Goals	Approach/Method/Experiment	Dataset/Sampling	Findings/Results
19	(Damen et al., 2018)	Determine the prevalence and antibiotic susceptibility of *S. aureus* nasal carriage among medical laboratory science students	Culture, gram and biochemical tests for identification of *S. aureus*. Disc diffusion performed for ABST	241 medical laboratory science students. Nasal swabs collected	A high prevalence of *S. aureus* nasal carriage noted
20	(Dunyach-Remy et al., 2017)	Compare genotypic profile of *S. aureus* strains isolated from nares and diabetic foot ulcers	Biochemical identification and antibiotic susceptibility of *S. aureus* by VITEK 2 automated system. Genotyping done with *S. aureus* genotyping kits	276 patients with diabetic foot ulcers. Nasal swabs and wound swabs collected	A high percentage of the diabetic population harbours the same *S. aureus* isolate in both wounds and nares.
21	(El Aila et al., 2017)	Prevalence of *S. aureus* and MRSA carriage among health care workers	Cross-sectional study. Organism identification by culture, gram and biochemical tests. ABST by disk diffusion. *mec*A gene detection by PCR	200 nasal swabs from health care workers	Nasal carriage of MRSA high among health care workers
22	(Nakamura et al., 2017)	Effect of nasal carriage of *S. aureus* on surgical site infection (SSI)	Statistical analysis identifying the significance of results	4148 patients screened for nasal bacterial carriage before orthopaedic surgery	Patients with nasal carriage of *S. aureus* had a higher incidence of SSI than those without.
23	(Walsh et al., 2018)	Determine if there is a specific patient population at increased risk of *S. aureus* nasal colonisation	Nasal screening is done six weeks before surgery and five days before surgery after chlorhexidine wash. Univariate and multivariate analysis to determine independent risk factors	716 patients undergoing primary or revision total hip arthroplasty (THA) and knee arthroplasty (TKA)	Patients on dialysis and patients with diabetes mellitus had a higher carrier rate of *S. aureus*
24	(Karabay, 2016)	Investigate and compare the frequency of nasal carriage of *S. aureus* in preclinical and clinical students	*S. aureus* identified by culture and biochemical testing. ABST did by disc diffusion	Nasal swabs were taken from 146 medical students; 82 preclinical and 64 clinical students	Frequency of nasal carriage of *S. aureus* four times higher in clinical than preclinical students
25	(Rampal et al., 2020)	Detect colonisation and contributory factors of MRSA on neckties, headscarves, and I.D. badges among medical students	Cross sectionals study. MRSA was identified using traditional culture and PCR.	251 students participated and 433 swab samples were collected from accessories	A significant association between preclinical vs. clinical medical students and *S. aureus* colonisation on neckties, headscarves, and ID badges

No.	Author, year	Purpose/Aims/Goals	Approach/Method/Experiment	Dataset/Sampling	Findings/Results
26	(Albert et al., 2018)	Determine the prevalence of *S. aureus* nasal colonisation in patients with rheumatoid arthritis (R.A.)	Detection of *S. aureus* by culturing and biochemical testing	Nasal swabs of 207 patients with rheumatoid arthritis and 37 healthy controls	No significant difference between R.A. patients and the general population in the prevalence of *S. aureus* nasal colonisation.
27	(Hobbs et al., 2018)	Determine the prevalence and risk factors of *S. aureus* colonisation and examine the association with the community-onset of infection	*S. aureus* identification by culture and MALDI-TOF mass spectrometry. ABST did by disk diffusion	5006 nasal swabs, 4868 oropharyngeal swabs, and 5105 skin swabs from a total of 5126 children	*S. aureus* colonisation is associated with community-onset of skin and soft tissue infections
28	(Haque et al., 2016)	Identify the knowledge level of medical students about antibiotic resistance in clinical years of university	Cross-sectional questionnaire-based survey.	164 students studying MBBS in years III, IV, and V	Identified that there is a gap between theoretical input and clinical practice
29	(Huang et al., 2019)	Nasal carriage of MRSA among international conference attendees	Detection of MRSA by PCR and cefoxitin disc. Genotyping and molecular characterisation by PFGE, MLST.	Nasal swabs of 209 conference attendees from 23 countries	MRSA carriage rates were similar to previous studies.
30	(Lin et al., 2020)	Assess the concordance between colonisation and clinical MRSA isolates	*S. aureus* identified by culture and biochemical testing. ABST by disc diffusion and E-test. For molecular characterisation, PFGE used	Nasal swabs of 354 diabetic patients, 112 with foot ulcer and 242 without foot ulcer	Nasal MRSA carriage is a significant risk factor for foot ulcer MRSA infection
31	(El-Mahdy et al., 2018)	Frequency of *S. aureus* and predominant clones including MRSA colonisation in the nares of healthy individuals	*S. aureus* identified by culture and biochemical testing. ABST by disc diffusion and molecular characterisation by PFGE, PCR, and MLST.	Two hundred ten healthy individuals; 70 non-hospitalised adults, 68 clinical students, 72 HCWS. Nasal swabs collected	Higher colonisation rate in the healthy community compared to clinical students and HCWs
32	(Bhoi et al., 2020)	Prevalence and risk factors for MRSA nasal colonisation in diabetic patients	Culture and biochemical testing for the identification of *S. aureus*. ABST by disc diffusion	Four hundred two patients were diagnosed with diabetes. Nasal swabs collected	Nasal colonisation rate of MRSA higher in diabetes mellitus patients
33	(Wu et al., 2019)	Prevalence of nasal carriage and diversity of MRSA among patients and HCWs	The mecA gene and cefoxitin resistance identify MRSA. ABST by disc diffusion.	Nasal swabs of 204 patients visiting the emergency department and 326 HCWS	Nasal MRSA colonisation was observed in both patients and HCWs

No.	Author, year	Purpose/Aims/Goals	Approach/Method/Experiment	Dataset/Sampling	Findings/Results
34	(Rasheed & Hussein, 2020)	Prevalence rate and antibiotic sensitivity profile of *S. aureus* in secondary school students	A cross-sectional community-based study. *S. aureus* identification by culture and biochemical.	Four hundred ninety-two students were selected based on exclusion criteria. Nasal	A high prevalence of *S. aureus* with increased antibiotic resistance was seen in the
			testing. ABST by disc diffusion	swabs were collected	selected population.
35	(Azmi et al., 2020)	Prevalence of *S. aureus* in the oral cavity of healthy adults	A cross-sectional study. Culture and biochemical testing were performed to identify *S. aureus*.	140 oral rinse samples from healthy individuals	High prevalence of *S. aureus* in the oral cavity of healthy adults
36	(Seow et al., 2021)	Identify the prevalence of *S. aureus* and its antimicrobial profile among food handlers	*S. aureus was* identified and antibiotic susceptibility testing done	200 hand swab samples from food handlers and 100 cooked food samples	Increased prevalence of *S. aureus* (95%) among food handlers including MDRSA
37	(Hanson et al., 2018)	Determine the prevalence of *S. aureus* colonisation in the nares and oropharynx of healthy persons and risk factors associated	*S. aureus* isolated and identified by culturing and biochemical testing. *mec*A, *nuc,* and 16S rRNA gene identified by PCR	Nasal and oropharyngeal swabs of 263 participants; 177 adults and 86 minors	Higher prevalence of *S. aureus* colonisation identified with the addition of oropharyngeal swab and environmental contamination known as the strongly associated risk factor
38	(Oberoi et al., 2020)	Detect inducible clindamycin resistance in nasal carriers of *S. aureus*	A prospective cross-sectional study. Identification of *S. aureus* by culture and biochemical testing and ABST by disc diffusion. D-test for detection of inducible clindamycin resistance	Nasal samples of 100 nursing staff and doctors	Increasing incidence of MRSA and inducible clindamycin resistance among health care workers
39	(Carrel et al., 2017)	Emergence and diffusion of clindamycin and erythromycin-resistant MSSA among veterans	A retrospective cohort was conducted to identify MSSA invasive infections. MSSA isolates tested against tetracycline, lincosamides, and macrolides only included	34,025 patient isolates meeting inclusion criteria included	Increase in phenotypic of potential ST398 (resistant to clindamycin and erythromycin but tetracycline susceptible) MSSA
40	(Che Hamzah et al., 2019)	Evaluate susceptibility profiles of MRSA and MSSA and determine the prevalence of inducible clindamycin resistance	ABST testing was performed by disc diffusion. Tigecycline and vancomycin resistance detected by MIC	199 *S. aureus* strains, 90 MRSA and 109 MSSA	Overall high prevalence of inducible clindamycin resistance and tigecycline resistance seen

Table 1.
Summary of studies on S. aureus isolated from healthy individuals from 2016 to 2020.

infective endocarditis among them. The study revealed that 16% of patients with SAB had confirmed infective endocarditis [80]. Also, *S. aureus* has been reported as the most frequent causative organism (29.4%) in hospitalised patients diagnosed with infective endocarditis in a Canadian study [81].

Numerous studies have demonstrated a significant incidence of *S. aureus* in healthcare settings that are resistant to antibiotics. There is, however, a significant difference between these studies and those that were carried out in community settings. This is due to the fact that little effort is made at the local level to address the global antibiotic resistance crisis, despite the fact that studies comparing the prevalence of antibiotic resistance in both communities and hospitals all showed consistently high values without a discernible difference. Influenced by many factors including crowded housing, poor cleanliness, inadequate access to healthcare, educational background and contact with asymptomatic MDRSA carriers are all typical causes of community-acquired diseases. Therefore, the evidence of the high incidence of *S. aureus* antibiotic resistance among healthy individuals from 2016 to 2020 has been prescribed in **Table 1**.

4. Antimicrobial resistance patterns

Antibiotic resistance is a huge global threat rising dangerously to a high level. According to the WHO global priority list of antibiotic-resistant bacteria, *S. aureus* is categorised as a priority 2 or level 'high' organism [82]. The emergence of antibiotic resistance among *S. aureus* dates back to the 1940s during which penicillin-resistant *S. aureus* was identified [14]. The penicillin-resistant *S. aureus* expressed a β-lactamase that hydrolysed the β-lactam ring found in antibiotics that target the cell wall [18].

The development of methicillin resistance among *S. aureus* isolates dates to the 1960s, increasing MRSA in hospital infections and later in community-acquired infections [5, 83]. Resistant to methicillin in *S. aureus* occurs by the expression of the methicillin-hydrolysing β-lactamase and a foreign penicillin-binding protein (PBP) [84]. The methicillin-resistant *S. aureus* differs from the methicillin-sensitive *S. aureus* by the presence of the *mec*A gene which encodes the PBP2a [85]. Hence, molecular characterisation of *S. aureus* is vital in identifying virulence genes such as Panton-valentine leucocidin (PVL) and the *mec*A gene responsible for antibiotic resistance of the organism [86].

The prevalence of MRSA among clinical isolates and community samples still exists [39, 40, 87], but recent studies reveal a decrease in MRSA prevalence specifically in the community [88–91]. To identify whether an MRSA isolate is community-associated or not molecular testing can be done to identify the presence of the gene SCCmec types IV and V as these two types are the most prevalent among CA-MRSA strains [89]. Similarly, *spa* typing to identify the *spa* gene of *S. aureus* helps in understanding the genetic diversity and clonal relatedness of the isolated organisms [92]. While the *spa* gene informs us of the presence of *S. aureus* in the specimen, its occurrence, together with the *mec*A gene, indicates the presence of MRSA [93]. Likewise, identifying the *scn* gene can suggest that the organism originated from livestock [94, 95].

With the decrease in the prevalence of MRSA seen in different populations, an increase in resistance to lincosamides and macrolides among *S. aureus* was identified [34, 96, 97]. Lincosamides are a class of antibiotics containing natural, lincomycin, and semi-synthetic chlorinated derivative clindamycin [98]. These antibiotics act by inhibiting protein synthesis and have good antibacterial activity against *Staphylococcus* and *Streptococcus* species and can suppress the expression of virulence factors in *S. aureus,* therefore, clindamycin is recommended for the treatment of toxin-mediated infections [99]. Macrolides, including erythromycin, are similar to lincosamides as their mechanism of action is by inhibiting protein synthesis and is effective in the treatment of Gram-positive organisms including *Staphylococcus* species [100]. However, recent studies raise the concern of increased clindamycin and erythromycin resistance seen among *S. aureus* isolates. *S. aureus* isolated from various clinical specimens from a hospital in Italy were subjected to antimicrobial susceptibility testing to identify the resistance rates and revealed the increase in resistance to clindamycin in sputum isolates (58.3%) and erythromycin in urine isolates (51.55%) [101]. Resistance to clindamycin is the result of enzymatic methylation of the antibiotic binding site of the ribosomal subunit [99]. The methylase is coded by a variety of *erm* genes of which *erm*A and *erm*C are found in *Staphylococcus* resulting in the production of rRNA methylase always (cMLS$_B$) or producing methylase only in the presence of an inducer (iMLS$_B$) such as erythromycin [102].

A study conducted among school children in Kathmandu, Nepal revealed 23.4% isolates to show inducible resistance to clindamycin [103]. Similarly 15.2% of isolates from clinical specimens from an Iran hospital showed inducible clindamycin resistance [104]. As both antimicrobial groups, namely lincosamides and macrolides, have been used to treat *S. aureus* infections in Malaysia since 2015 [22], identifying the resistance pattern for these antibiotics is deemed necessary. A study conducted among health care workers of a tertiary hospital in Terengganu, Malaysia, highlighted the increase in the prevalence of inducible clindamycin resistance and tigecycline resistance among MRSA and MSSA isolates from nasal samples of health care workers [105].

5. Multidrug-Resistant *S. aureus*

Replace *S. aureus* is known to have the ability to quickly develop resistance to each new antibiotic that is used [106]. Various mechanisms adapted by *S. aureus* include inactivating the antibiotic, altering the target of antibiotic, use of efflux pumps to reduce the intake of antibiotics and trapping the antibiotic [106]. A bacterium is regarded as a multidrug-resistant organism when it becomes resistant to more than one antibiotic either by having several different resistant genes or a single resistance mechanism providing resistance to more than one antibiotic [107]. Multidrug-resistant *S. aureus* is a huge problem in hospital settings as well as in the community. For *S. aureus* when the organism is identified as an MRSA it is regarded as a multidrug-resistant (MDR) to oxacillin or cefoxitin renders the organism non-susceptible to all types of β-lactams, including cephalosporins, penicillin's, β-lactamase inhibitors and carbapenems [108]. Increased resistance to antibiotics was identified among MRSA strains in a study conducted in Taiwan and China [109]. Three hundred and thirty-two strains of MRSA were included from the two countries which showed increased resistance to chloramphenicol (43%) and trimethoprim-sulfamethoxazole (89.0%). A study conducted in India with 783 strains of *S. aureus* from different clinical specimens revealed 301 (38.4%) MRSA out of which 72.1% were multidrug-resistant. Among these MDR strains, 136 were resistant to more than three antimicrobial groups

Apart from methicillin resistance in *S. aureus*, resistance to agents such as linezolid's, vancomycin and teicoplanin and daptomycin has also been reported [110]. Vancomycin-resistant *S. aureus* (VRSA) strains have now been documented globally since the first clinical isolate was discovered in 1997 [111–113]. The VRSA prevalence increased by 3.5 times between the years before to 2006 and 2020, from 2% in the pre-2006 period to 5% in the 2006–2014 period to 7% in the post–2015 period [114].

6. Conclusion

This chapter offers more proof of the significant incidence of multidrug-resistant *S. aureus* in community settings, coming from healthy human sources. These findings should motivate those involved in health research, medicine, advocacy organisations, and health policymakers to collaborate in order to create effective solutions to address this growing global health problem. In order to stop the spread of resistance, it is urgently advised that community-level methods similar to those used in clinical settings, such as monitoring, awareness-raising, improved sanitation and hygiene, prompt disease diagnosis, and strict prescription regulations, be put into place.

Author details

Asdren Zajmi[1]*, Fathimath Shiranee[2], Shirley Gee Hoon Tang[3], Mohammed A.M. Alhoot[2] and Sairah Abdul Karim[2]

1 Faculty of Health and Life Sciences, Management and Science University, Shah Alam, Selangor, Malaysia

2 Post Graduate Centre, Management and Science University, Shah Alam, Selangor, Malaysia

3 Center for Toxicology and Health Risk Studies (CORE), Faculty of Health Sciences, Universiti Kebangsaan Malaysia, Jalan Raja Muda Abdul Aziz, Kuala Lumpur, Malaysia

*Address all correspondence to: asdren_zajmi@msu.edu.my

References

[1] Taylor TA, Unakal CG. *Staphylococcus aureus*. In: StatPearls [Internet]. Treasure Island (FL): StatPearls Publishing; 2022

[2] Nandhini P, Kumar P, Mickymaray S, Alothaim AS, Somasundaram J, Rajan M. Recent developments in methicillin-resistant Staphylococcus aureus (MRSA) treatment: A review. Antibiotics (Basel). 2022;**11**(5):606

[3] Ambachew A, Gebrecherkos T, Ayalew G. Prevalence and clindamycin resistance profile of Staphylococcus aureus and associated factors among patients attending the University of Gondar Comprehensive Specialized Hospital, Gondar, Northwest Ethiopia. Interdisciplinary Perspectives on Infectious Diseases. 2022;**2022**:1-10

[4] Krismer B, Weidenmaier C, Zipperer A, Peschel A. The commensal lifestyle of Staphylococcus aureus and its interactions with the nasal microbiota. Nature Reviews Microbiology. 2017;**15**(11):675-687

[5] Lee AS, De Lencastre H, Garau J, Kluytmans J, Malhotra-Kumar S, Peschel A, et al. Methicillin-resistant *Staphylococcus aureus*. Nature Reviews Disease Primers. 2018;**4**(1):1-23

[6] Duarte FC, Danelli T, Tavares ER, Morguette AEB, Kerbauy G, Grion CMC, et al. Fatal sepsis caused by mecA-positive oxacillin-susceptible *Staphylococcus aureus*: First report in a tertiary hospital of southern Brazil. Journal of Infection and Chemotherapy. 2019;**25**(4):293-297

[7] de Oliveira CF, Morey AT, Santos JP, Gomes LV, Cardoso JD, Pinge-Filho P, et al. Molecular and phenotypic characteristics of methicillin-resistant *Staphylococcus aureus* isolated from hospitalized patients. Journal of Infection in Developing Countries. 2015;**9**(7):743-751

[8] Hamdan-Partida A, Sainz-Espuñes T, Bustos-Martínez J. Characterization and persistence of *Staphylococcus aureus* strains isolated from the anterior nares and throats of healthy carriers in a Mexican community. Journal of Clinical Microbiology. 2010;**48**(5):1701-1705

[9] Hamdan-Partida A, González-García S, de la Rosa García E, Bustos-Martínez J. Community-acquired methicillin-resistant *Staphylococcus aureus* can persist in the throat. International Journal of Medical Microbiology. 2018;**308**(4):469-475

[10] González-García S, Hamdan-Partida A, Bustos-Hamdan A, Bustos-Martínez J. Factors of nasopharynx that favor the colonization and persistence of *Staphylococcus aureus*. In: Zhou ZZX, editor. Pharynx-Diagnosis and Treatment. London, UK., London, UK: IntechOpen; 2021. pp. 163-180

[11] Pollitt EJG, Szkuta PT, Burns N, Foster SJ. *Staphylococcus aureus* infection dynamics. PLoS Pathogens. 2018;**14**(6):e1007112

[12] Sakr A, Bregeon F, Mege JL, Rolain JM, Blin O. *Staphylococcus aureus* nasal colonization: An update on mechanisms, epidemiology, risk factors, and subsequent infections. Frontiers in Microbiology. 2018;**9**:2419

[13] Ryan KJ. Sherris medical microbiology. In: Staphylococci. McGraw-Hill; 2017

[14] Chambers HF, Deleo FR. Waves of resistance: *Staphylococcus aureus*

in the antibiotic era. Nature Reviews Microbiology. 2009;7(9):629-641

[15] Paling FP, Wolkewitz M, Bode LG, Klouwenberg PK, Ong DS, Depuydt P, et al. *Staphylococcus aureus* colonization at ICU admission as a risk factor for developing S. aureus ICU pneumonia. Clinical Microbiology and Infection. 2017;**23**(1):49. e9-49. e14

[16] Young BC, Wu CH, Gordon NC, Cole K, Price JR, Liu E, et al. Severe infections emerge from commensal bacteria by adaptive evolution. eLife. 2017;**6**:e30637

[17] Rammelkamp CH, Maxon T. Resistance of *Staphylococcus aureus* to the action of penicillin. Experimental Biology and Medicine. 1942;**51**(3):386-389

[18] Foster TJ. Antibiotic resistance in *Staphylococcus aureus*. Current status and future prospects. FEMS Microbiology Reviews. 2017;**41**(3):430-449

[19] Mendelson M, Sharland M, Mpundu M. Antibiotic resistance: Calling time on the 'silent pandemic'. JAC-Antimicrobial Resistance. 2022;**4**(2):dlac016

[20] Qiao Y, Ning X, Chen Q, Zhao R, Song W, Zheng Y, et al. Clinical and molecular characteristics of invasive community-acquired *Staphylococcus aureus* infections in Chinese children. BMC Infectious Diseases. 2014;**14**(1):1-10

[21] Ragbetli C, Parlak M, Bayram Y, Guducuoglu H, Ceylan N. Evaluation of antimicrobial resistance in *Staphylococcus aureus* isolates by years. Interdisciplinary Perspectives on Infectious Diseases. 2016;**2016**:9171395

[22] Hamzah AMC, Yeo CC, Puah SM, Chua KH, Rahman NIA, Abdullah FH, et al. Tigecycline and inducible clindamycin resistance in clinical isolates of methicillin-resistant *Staphylococcus aureus* from Terengganu, Malaysia. Journal of Medical Microbiology. 2019;**68**(9):1299-1305

[23] Wang X, Shen Y, Huang W, Zhou Y. Characterisation of community-acquired *Staphylococcus aureus* causing skin and soft tissue infections in a children's hospital in Shanghai, China. Epidemiology and Infection. 2019;**147**:e323

[24] Chinnambedu RS, Marimuthu RR, Sunil SS, Amrose P, Ramachandran V, Pachamuthu B. Changing antibiotic resistance profile of *Staphylococcus aureus* isolated from HIV patients (2012-2017) in southern India. Journal of Infection and Public Health. 2020;**13**(1):75-79

[25] Rossato AM, Primon-Barros M, Rocha LdL, Reiter KC, Dias CAG, d'Azevedo PA. Resistance profile to antimicrobials agents in methicillin-resistant *Staphylococcus aureus* isolated from hospitals in South Brazil between 2014-2019. Revista da Sociedade Brasileira de Medicina Tropical. 2020:53

[26] Stryjewski ME, Chambers HF. Skin and soft-tissue infections caused by community-acquired methicillin-resistant *Staphylococcus aureus*. Clinical Infectious Diseases. 2008;**46**(Suppl. 5 (Supplement_5)):S368-S377

[27] Cameron JK, Hall L, Tong SY, Paterson DL, Halton K. Incidence of community onset MRSA in Australia: Least reported where it is Most prevalent. Antimicrobial Resistance & Infection Control. 2019;**8**(1):1-9

[28] Junnila J, Hirvioja T, Rintala E, Auranen K, Rantakokko-Jalava K, Silvola J, et al. Changing epidemiology of methicillin-resistant *Staphylococcus aureus* in a low endemicity

area-new challenges for MRSA control. European Journal of Clinical Microbiology & Infectious Diseases. 2020;**39**(12):2299-2307

[29] Petersen A, Larssen KW, Gran FW, Enger H, Haeggman S, Makitalo B, et al. Increasing incidences and clonal diversity of methicillin-resistant *Staphylococcus aureus* in the Nordic countries - results from the Nordic MRSA surveillance. Future Microbiology. 2021;**12**:668900

[30] Chen CJ, Huang YC. New epidemiology of *Staphylococcus aureus* infection in Asia. Clinical Microbiology and Infection. 2014;**20**(7):605-623

[31] Shaw AG, Vento TJ, Mende K, Kreft RE, Ehrlich GD, Wenke JC, et al. Detection of methicillin-resistant and methicillin-susceptible *Staphylococcus aureus* colonization of healthy military personnel by traditional culture, PCR, and mass spectrometry. Scandinavian Journal of Infectious Diseases. 2013;**45**(10):752-759

[32] Tigabu A, Tiruneh M, Mekonnen F. Nasal Carriage Rate, Antimicrobial Susceptibility Pattern, and Associated Factors of *Staphylococcus aureus* with Special Emphasis on MRSA among Urban and Rural Elementary School Children in Gondar. Northwest Ethiopia: A comparative cross-sectional study. Advances in Preventive Medicine; 2018. p. 2018

[33] Yan X, Song Y, Yu X, Tao X, Yan J, Luo F, et al. Factors associated with *Staphylococcus aureus* nasal carriage among healthy people in northern China. Clinical Microbiology and Infection. 2015;**21**(2):157-162

[34] Suhaili Z, Azis NM, Yeo CC, Nordin SA, Rahim ARA, Al-Obaidi MMJ, et al. Characterization of resistance to selected antibiotics and Panton-valentine leukocidin-positive *Staphylococcus aureus* in a healthy student population at a Malaysian university. GERMS. 2018;**8**(1):21

[35] Brown AF, Leech JM, Rogers TR, McLoughlin RM. *Staphylococcus aureus* colonization: Modulation of Host immune response and impact on human vaccine design. Frontiers in Immunology. 2014;**4**:507

[36] Hanssen AM, Kindlund B, Stenklev NC, Furberg AS, Fismen S, Olsen RS, et al. Localization of *Staphylococcus aureus* in tissue from the nasal vestibule in healthy carriers. BMC Microbiology. 2017;**17**(1):89

[37] Ucuncu H, Uslu H, Ozbek A, Aktan B, Sutbeyaz Y, Altas E. Comparison of the bacterial flora of the nasal vestibule and cavity in haemodialysis patients. Acta Otorhinolaryngologica Italica. 2009;**29**(5):251-254

[38] Nouwen JL, Ott A, Kluytmans-Vandenbergh MF, Boelens HA, Hofman A, Van Belkum A, et al. Predicting the *Staphylococcus aureus* nasal carrier state: Derivation and validation of a "culture rule". Clinical Infectious Diseases. 2004;**39**(6):806-811

[39] Ansari S, Gautam R, Shrestha S, Ansari SR, Subedi SN, Chhetri MR. Risk factors assessment for nasal colonization of *Staphylococcus aureus* and its methicillin resistant strains among pre-clinical medical students of Nepal. BMC Research Notes. 2016;**9**(1):1-8

[40] Chen B, Xie X, Ni L, Dai X, Lu Y, Wu X, et al. Factors associated with *Staphylococcus aureus* nasal carriage and molecular characteristics among the general population at a medical college campus in Guangzhou, South China. Annals of Clinical Microbiology and Antimicrobials. 2017;**16**(1):1-10

[41] Ahmadi E, Khojasteh M, Mortazavi SM, Khan-Mohammadi F, Kazemnia A, Beheshtipour J, et al. Prevalence of and risk factors for methicillin-resistant *Staphylococcus aureus* nasal carriage in the west of Iran: A population-based cross-sectional study. BMC Infectious Diseases. 2019;**19**(1):1-8

[42] Conceição T, Martins H, Rodrigues S, de Lencastre H, Aires-de-Sousa M. *Staphylococcus aureus* nasal carriage among homeless population in Lisbon, Portugal. European Journal of Clinical Microbiology & Infectious Diseases. 2019;**38**(11):2037-2044

[43] El-Mahdy TS, Al-Agamy MH, Emara M, Barakat A, Goering RV. Complex clonal diversity of *Staphylococcus aureus* nasal colonization among community personnel, healthcare workers, and clinical students in the Eastern Province, Saudi Arabia. BioMed Research International. 2018;**2018**

[44] Hanson BM, Kates AE, O'Malley SM, Mills E, Herwaldt LA, Torner JC, et al. *Staphylococcus aureus* in the nose and throat of Iowan families. Epidemiology and Infection. 2018;**146**(14):1777-1784

[45] Azmi AH, Adnan SNA, Ab Malik N. Thc prevalence of *Staphylococcus aureus* in the Oral cavity of healthy adults in Malaysia. Sains Malaysiana. 2020;**49**(3):583-591

[46] Muenks CE, Hogan PG, Wang JW, Eisenstein KA, Burnham C-AD, Fritz SA. Diversity of *Staphylococcus aureus* strains colonizing various niches of the human body. Journal of Infection. 2016;**72**(6):698-705

[47] Nakamura M, Shimakawa T, Nakano S, Chikawa T, Yoshioka S, Kashima M, et al. Screening for nasal carriage of *Staphylococcus aureus* among patients scheduled to undergo orthopedic surgery: Incidence of surgical site infection by nasal carriage. Journal of Orthopaedic Science. 2017;**22**(4):778-782

[48] Bhoi P, Otta S, Swain B, Kar BR. Prevalence of nasal carriage of MRSA in diabetic patients attending the outpatient department. International Journal of Research in Medical Sciences. 2020;**8**(4):1336

[49] Lin S-Y, Lin N-Y, Huang Y-Y, Hsieh C-C, Huang Y-C. Methicillin-resistant *Staphylococcus aureus* nasal carriage and infection among patients with diabetic foot ulcer. Journal of Microbiology, Immunology and Infection. 2020;**53**(2):292-299

[50] Walsh ALF, Adam C, Dieterich JD, Chen DD, Bronson MJ, Moucha CS. Risk factors for *Staphylococcus aureus* nasal colonization in joint replacement patients. The Journal of Arthroplasty. 2018;**33**(5):1530-1533

[51] Hidron AI, Kempker R, Moanna A, Rimland D. Methicillin-resistant *Staphylococcus aureus* in HIV-infected patients. Infection and Drug Resistance. 2010;**3**:73-86

[52] Kotpal R, Bhalla P, Dewan R, Kaur R. Incidence and risk factors of nasal carriage of *Staphylococcus aureus* in HIV-infected individuals in comparison to HIV-uninfected individuals: A case-control study. Journal of the International Association of Providers of AIDS Care (JIAPAC). 2016;**15**(2):141-147

[53] Olsen K, Danielsen K, Wilsgaard T, Sangvik M, Sollid JU, Thune I, et al. Obesity and *Staphylococcus aureus* nasal colonization among women and men in a general population. PLoS One. 2013;**8**(5):e63716

[54] Albert G, Ricse M, Narvaez J, Rodriguez-Moreno J, Nolla JM, Dominguez-Luzon M, et al. Prevalence of nasal colonization with *Staphylococcus aureus* in patients with rheumatoid arthritis. Current Rheumatology Reviews. 2018;**14**(1):78-83

[55] Wang H-K, Huang C-Y, Chen C-J, Huang Y-C. Nasal *Staphylococcus aureus* and methicillin-resistant *Staphylococcus aureus* carriage among college student athletes in northern Taiwan. Journal of Microbiology, Immunology and Infection. 2017;**50**(4):537-540

[56] Kadariya J, Thapaliya D, Bhatta S, Mahatara RL, Bempah S, Dhakal N, et al. Multidrug-resistant *Staphylococcus aureus* colonization in healthy adults is more common in Bhutanese refugees in Nepal than those resettled in Ohio. BioMed Research International. 2019;**2019**

[57] Curry JA, Maguire JD, Fraser J, Tribble DR, Deiss RG, Bryan C, et al. Prevalence of *Staphylococcus aureus* colonization and risk factors for infection among military personnel in a shipboard setting. Military Medicine. 2016;**181**(6):524-529

[58] Tacconelli E, De Angelis G, Cataldo MA, Pozzi E, Cauda R. Does antibiotic exposure increase the risk of methicillin-resistant *Staphylococcus aureus* (MRSA) isolation? A systematic review and meta-analysis. Journal of Antimicrobial Chemotherapy. 2008;**61**(1):26-38

[59] Wooten D, Winston L. Risk factors for methicillin-resistant *Staphylococcus aureus* in patients with community-onset and hospital-onset pneumonia. Respiratory Medicine. 2013;**107**(8):1266-1270

[60] Wong J, Siti-Azrin A, Mohd-Fadhli K, Siti-Asma H. Low prevalence of *Staphylococcus aureus* colonization among dental students in a teaching hospital in Malaysia. Tropical Biomedicine. 2018;**35**(1):246-251

[61] Rampal S, Zainuddin NH, Elias NA, Tengku Jamaluddin TZM, Maniam S, Teh SW, et al. Colonization of methicillin-resistant *Staphylococcus aureus* (MRSA) among medical students in tertiary institution in Central Malaysia. Antibiotics. 2020;**9**(7):382

[62] Seow W-L, Mahyudin NA, Amin-Nordin S, Radu S, Abdul-Mutalib NA. Antimicrobial resistance of *Staphylococcus aureus* among cooked food and food handlers associated with their occupational information in Klang Valley, Malaysia. Food Control. 2021;**124**:107872

[63] Ukpanah MA, Upla PU. Why is *Staphylococcus aureus* such a successful pathogen? Microbiology Research Journal International. 2017;**19**:1-22

[64] Gnanamani A, Hariharan P, Paul-Satyaseela M. *Staphylococcus aureus*: Overview of bacteriology, clinical diseases, epidemiology, antibiotic resistance and therapeutic approach. Frontiers in *Staphylococcus aureus*. 2017;**4**(28):10.5772

[65] Stygall J, Newman S. Hospital acquired Anfection. In: Cambridge Handbook of Psychology, Health and Medicine. Cambridge, UK: Cambridge University Press; 2014. pp. 736-738

[66] Tolera M, Abate D, Dheresa M, Marami D. Bacterial nosocomial infections and antimicrobial susceptibility pattern among patients admitted at Hiwot Fana specialized university hospital, eastern Ethiopia. Advances in Medicine. 2018;**2018**

[67] Nimer NA. Nosocomial infection and antibiotic-resistant threat in the Middle

East. Infection and Drug Resistance. 2022;**15**:631-639

[68] Doudoulakakis A, Spiliopoulou I, Giormezis N, Syridou G, Nika A, Bozavoutoglou E, et al. Methicillin-resistant *Staphylococcus aureus* transmission and hospital-acquired bacteremia in a neonatal intensive care unit in Greece. Journal of Infection and Chemotherapy. 2022;**28**(2):176-180

[69] Idris S, Rukumani D, Nadia A, Ra AR. A descriptive study on bacterial Aetiology of ventilator-associated pneumonia in Sungai Buloh hospital, Malaysia. International Journal of Public Health and Clinical Sciences. 2022;**9**(2):1-8

[70] Bloomfield LE, Coombs GW, Tempone S, Armstrong PK. Marked increase in community-associated methicillin-resistant *Staphylococcus aureus* infections, Western Australia, 2004-2018. Epidemiology and Infection. 2020;**148**:e153

[71] Yamaguchi T, Nakamura I, Sato T, Ono D, Sato A, Sonoda S, et al. Changes in the genotypic characteristics of community-acquired methicillin-resistant Staphylococcus aureus collected in 244 medical facilities in Japan between 2010 and 2018: A Nationwide surveillance. Microbiology Spectrum. 2022:e02272-e02221

[72] Giormezis N, Doudoulakakis A, Tsilipounidaki K, Militsopoulou M, Kalogeras G, Stamouli V, et al. Emergence of a mupirocin-resistant, methicillin-susceptible *Staphylococcus aureus* clone associated with skin and soft tissue infections in Greece. BMC Microbiology. 2021;**21**(1):203

[73] Landrum ML, Neumann C, Cook C, Chukwuma U, Ellis MW, Hospenthal DR, et al. Epidemiology of *Staphylococcus aureus* blood and skin and soft tissue infections in the US military health system, 2005-2010. JAMA. 2012;**308**(1):50-59

[74] Kumar N, David MZ, Boyle-Vavra S, Sieth J, Daum RS. High *Staphylococcus aureus* colonization prevalence among patients with skin and soft tissue infections and controls in an urban emergency department. Journal of Clinical Microbiology. 2015;**53**(3):810-815

[75] Rimoldi SG, Pileri P, Mazzocco MI, Romeri F, Bestetti G, Calvagna N, et al. The role of *Staphylococcus aureus* in mastitis : A multidisciplinary working group experience. Journal of Human Lactation. 2020;**36**(3):503-509

[76] Tao YN, Tong XK, Qian C, Wan H, Zuo JP. Microbial quantitation of colostrum from healthy breastfeeding women and milk from mastitis patients. Annals of Palliative Medicine. 2020;**9**(4):1666-1680

[77] Smith JT, Eckhardt EM, Hansel NB, Eliato TR, Martin IW, Andam CP. Genomic epidemiology of methicillin-resistant and - susceptible *Staphylococcus aureus* from bloodstream infections. BMC Infectious Diseases. 2021;**21**(1):589

[78] Marra AR, Camargo LF, Pignatari AC, Sukiennik T, Behar PR, Medeiros EA, et al. Nosocomial bloodstream infections in Brazilian hospitals: Analysis of 2,563 cases from a prospective nationwide surveillance study. Journal of Clinical Microbiology. 2011;**49**(5):1866-1871

[79] Grundmann H, Schouls LM, Aanensen DM, Pluister GN, Tami A, Chlebowicz M, et al. European staphylococcal reference laboratory working, the dynamic changes of dominant clones of *Staphylococcus aureus*

causing bloodstream infections in the European region: Results of a second structured survey. Euro Surveillance. 2014;**19**(49):20987

[80] Rasmussen RV, Host U, Arpi M, Hassager C, Johansen HK, Korup E, et al. Prevalence of infective endocarditis in patients with *Staphylococcus aureus* bacteraemia: The value of screening with echocardiography. European Journal of Echocardiography. 2011;**12**(6):414-420

[81] Mackie AS, Liu W, Savu A, Marelli AJ, Kaul P. Infective endocarditis hospitalizations before and after the 2007 American Heart Association prophylaxis guidelines. Canadian Journal of Cardiology. 2016;**32**(8):942-948

[82] Tacconelli E, Carrara E, Savoldi A, Harbarth S, Mendelson M, Monnet DL, et al. Discovery, research, and development of new antibiotics: The WHO priority list of antibiotic-resistant bacteria and tuberculosis. The Lancet Infectious Diseases. 2018;**18**(3):318-327

[83] Harkins CP, Pichon B, Doumith M, Parkhill J, Westh H, Tomasz A, et al. Methicillin-resistant *Staphylococcus aureus* emerged long before the introduction of methicillin into clinical practice. Genome Biology. 2017;**18**(1):1-11

[84] Stapleton PD, Taylor PW. Methicillin resistance in *Staphylococcus aureus*: Mechanisms and modulation. Science Progress. 2002;**85**(Pt 1):57-72

[85] Wielders C, Fluit A, Brisse S, Verhoef J, Schmitz F. mecA gene is widely disseminated in *Staphylococcus aureus* population. Journal of Clinical Microbiology. 2002;**40**(11):3970-3975

[86] Sabbagh P, Ebrahimzadeh-Namvar A, Ferdosi-Shahandashti E, Javanian M, Khafri S, Rajabnia M. Molecularcharacterizationof*Staphylococcus aureus* strains isolated among hospital staff nasal carriers of Babol, Iran. Caspian Journal of Internal Medicine. 2017;**8**(4):311

[87] Abroo S, Jazani NH, Sharifi Y. Methicillin-resistant *Staphylococcus aureus* nasal carriage between healthy students of medical and nonmedical universities. American Journal of Infection Control. 2017;**45**(7):709-712

[88] Okamo B, Moremi N, Seni J, Mirambo MM, Kidenya BR, Mshana SE. Prevalence and antimicrobial susceptibility profiles of *Staphylococcus aureus* nasal carriage among pre-clinical and clinical medical students in a Tanzanian university. BMC Research Notes. 2016;**9**(1):1-6

[89] Laub K, Tothpál A, Kovács E, Sahin-Tóth J, Horváth A, Kardos S, et al. High prevalence of *Staphylococcus aureus* nasal carriage among children in Szolnok, Hungary. Acta Microbiologica et Immunologica Hungarica. 2018;**65**(1):59-72

[90] Miragaia M. Factors contributing to the evolution of mecA-mediated beta-lactam resistance in staphylococci: Update and new insights from whole genome sequencing (WGS). Frontiers in Microbiology. 2018;**9**:2723

[91] Azis NM, Pung HP, Rachman ARA, Nordin SA, Sarchio SN, Suhaili Z, et al. A persistent antimicrobial resistance pattern and limited methicillin-resistance-associated genotype in a short-term *Staphylococcus aureus* carriage isolated from a student population. Journal of Infection and Public Health. 2017;**10**(2):156-164

[92] Goudarzi M, Fazeli M, Goudarzi H, Azad M, Seyedjavadi SS. Spa typing of *Staphylococcus aureus* strains isolated

from clinical specimens of patients with nosocomial infections in Tehran, Iran. Jundishapur Journal of Microbiology. 2016;**9**(7):e35685

[93] Le T-T, Nadimpalli M, Wu J, Heaney CD, Stewart JR. Challenges in estimating characteristics of *Staphylococcus aureus* nasal carriage among humans enrolled in surveillance studies. Frontiers in Public Health. 2018;**6**:163

[94] Stegger M, Liu CM, Larsen J, Soldanova K, Aziz M, Contente-Cuomo T, et al. Rapid differentiation between livestock-associated and livestock-independent *Staphylococcus aureus* CC398 clades. PLoS One. 2013;**8**(11):e79645

[95] Nadimpalli M, Rinsky JL, Wing S, Hall D, Stewart J, Larsen J, et al. Persistence of livestock-associated antibiotic-resistant *Staphylococcus aureus* among industrial hog operation workers in North Carolina over 14 days. Occupational and Environmental Medicine. 2015;**72**(2):90-99

[96] Carrel M, Goto M, Schweizer ML, David MZ, Livorsi D, Perencevich EN. Diffusion of clindamycin-resistant and erythromycin-resistant methicillin-susceptible *Staphylococcus aureus* (MSSA), potential ST398, in United States veterans health administration hospitals, 2003-2014. Antimicrobial Resistance & Infection Control. 2017;**6**(1):55

[97] Bidani J, Oberoi L, Malhotra A, Sidhu SK, Soneja S. Detection of inducible clindamycin resistance in nasal carriers of *Staphylococcus aureus* among healthcare workers. IP International Journal of Medical Microbiology Tropical Diseases. 2020;**6**(2)

[98] Spizek J, Rezanka T. Lincosamides: Chemical structure, biosynthesis, mechanism of action, resistance, and applications. Biochemical Pharmacology. 2017;**133**:20-28

[99] Hodille E, Badiou C, Bouveyron C, Bes M, Tristan A, Vandenesch F, et al. Clindamycin suppresses virulence expression in inducible clindamycin-resistant *Staphylococcus aureus* strains. Annals of Clinical Microbiology and Antimicrobials. 2018;**17**(1):38

[100] Dinos GP. The macrolide antibiotic renaissance. British Journal of Pharmacology. 2017;**174**(18):2967-2983

[101] Ronga L, Abbasciano A, Calia C, Mosca A, Battista M, Sparapano E, et al. Trends in the antibiotic resistance of S. aureus clinical isolates: A 4 years retrospective study in a teaching hospital in South Italy. Le Infezioni in Medicina. 2019;**27**(3):266-273

[102] Seifi N, Kahani N, Askari E, Mahdipour S, Naderi NM. Inducible clindamycin resistance in *Staphylococcus aureus* isolates recovered from Mashhad, IRan. Iranian Journal of Microbiology. 2012;**4**(2):82-86

[103] Timsina R, Shrestha U, Singh A, Timalsina B. Inducible clindamycin resistance and erm genes in *Staphylococcus aureus* in school children in Kathmandu, Nepa. Future Science OA. 2020;**7**(1):FSO361

[104] Baral R, Khanal B. Inducible clindamycin resistance in *Staphylococcus aureus* strains isolated from clinical samples. International Journal of Biomedical Research. 2017;**8**(2):81-84

[105] Che Hamzah AM, Yeo CC, Puah SM, Chua KH, Chew CH. *Staphylococcus aureus* infections in Malaysia: A review of antimicrobial resistance and characteristics of the clinical

isolates, 1990-2017. Antibiotics (Basel). 2019;**8**(3):128

[106] Pantosti A, Sanchini A, Monaco M. Mechanisms of antibiotic resistance in *Staphylococcus aureus*. Future Microbiology. 2007;**2**(3):323-334

[107] Gall E, Long A, Hall KK. Infections due to other multidrug-resistant organisms. In: Making Healthcare Safer III: A Critical Analysis of Existing and Emerging Patient Safety Practices [Internet]. USA: Agency for Healthcare Research and Quality (US); 2020

[108] Kaur DC, Chate SS. Study of antibiotic resistance pattern in methicillin resistant *Staphylococcus aureus* with special reference to newer antibiotic. Journal of Global Infectious Diseases. 2015;**7**(2):78-84

[109] Aires de Sousa M, Crisostomo MI, Sanches IS, Wu JS, Fuzhong J, Tomasz A, et al. Frequent recovery of a single clonal type of multidrug-resistant *Staphylococcus aureus* from patients in two hospitals in Taiwan and China. Journal of Clinical Microbiology. 2003;**41**(1):159-163

[110] Traczewski MM, Katz BD, Steenbergen JN, Brown SD. Inhibitory and bactericidal activities of daptomycin, vancomycin, and teicoplanin against methicillin-resistant *Staphylococcus aureus* isolates collected from 1985 to 2007. Antimicrobial Agents and Chemotherapy. 2009;**53**(5):1735-1738

[111] Afshari A, Taheri S, Hashemi M, Norouzy A, Nematy M, Mohamadi S. Methicillin-and vancomycin-resistant *Staphylococcus aureus* and vancomycin-resistant enterococci isolated from hospital foods: Prevalence and antimicrobial resistance patterns. Current Microbiology. 2022;**79**(11):1-10

[112] Hiramatsu K. Vancomycin-resistant *Staphylococcus aureus*: A new model of antibiotic resistance. The Lancet Infectious Diseases. 2001;**1**(3):147-155

[113] Eidaroos NH, Youssef AI, El-Sebae A, Enany ME, Farid DS. Genotyping of enterotoxigenic methicillin-resistant *Staphylococcus aureus* (MRSA) and vancomycin-resistant *Staphylococcus aureus* (VRSA) among commensal rodents in North Sinai, Egypt. Journal of Applied Microbiology. 2022;**132**(3):2331-2341

[114] Wu Q, Sabokroo N, Wang Y, Hashemian M, Karamollahi S, Kouhsari E. Systematic review and meta-analysis of the epidemiology of vancomycin-resistance *Staphylococcus aureus* isolates. Antimicrobial Resistance & Infection Control. 2021;**10**(1):1-13

Section 2

Epidemiology and Pathogenesis

Chapter 3

The Molecular Epidemiological Study of MRSA in Mexico

Miguel Ángel Ortíz Gil and Monica Irasu Cardona Alvarado

Abstract

The rapid spread of infections by methicillin-resistant *Staphylococcus aureus* (MRSA) emerged in the early 1960s, and this pathogen is one of the most common agents of nosocomial infections. As a reaction to the appearance and spread of multi-drug-resistant MRSA in Mexico, some hospitals have established molecular epidemiological surveillance, where pandemic clones of MRSA have been detected in different states in the north, the center, and the south of Mexico. The pandemic clones detected in Mexico are the Iberian, the New York/Japan, the pediatric, the EMRSA-16, and the USA-300. The surveillance or evolutionary studies carried out in Mexico, using different molecular methodologies, have shown a predominance of the New York/Japan clone, which has even displaced other MRSA clones. Therefore, it is necessary to continue establishing molecular surveillance and diagnostic programs as a special management for the confirmed MRSA infections, if these measures are not carried out to understand and control the changing lineages of MRSA, in the future, it may become an important public health problem, since the New York/Japan clone, which is the most predominant in our country, clearly demonstrates its great capacity for geographical expansion, multi-resistance, and virulence.

Keywords: *Staphylococcus aureus*, MRSA, clones, CA-MRSA, HA-MRSA, Mexico

1. Introduction

In Mexico, la Red Hospitalaria de Vigilancia Epidemiologica (RHVE) reported that mortality rates among patients infected with *S. aureus* show a variability between 5 and 70%, in addition to high attributable mortality rates, approximately 50% [1]. *S. aureus* produces a wide variety of exoproteins that contribute to its ability to colonize and cause disease in humans [2]. MRSA strains are characterized by the presence of a mobile genetic element called the staphylococcal cassette cromosoma *mec (SCCmec)*, which includes the *mecA* gene [3]. The structural *mecA* gene codes for penicillin-binding protein (PBP) 2a, which determines resistance to methicillin [4]. Modifications in PBP2a prevent PBP-penicillin binding, causing cell wall synthesis to proceed normally [5].

Nosocomial infections (NI) are considered a public health problem worldwide. For example, in the Latin American region, the SENTRY Surveillance Antimicrobial Program reported an increase in the proportion of MRSA in medical centers from

33.8% in 1997 to 40.2% in 2006. In Mexico, some studies show an increase in the prevalence of MRSA in recent years, and the incidence of NI ranges between 3.8 and 26.1 cases per 100 discharges; mortality associated with nosocomial infections is an average of 5%, and in 2001, it was the seventh leading cause of death for the general population in 2001 [6]. Reports from the Pan American Health Organization (PAHO) for Mexico informed that there was a prevalence of 52% of MRSA in 2004, while the Pan American Association of Infectious Diseases reported 32% in 2006, and data from the study of the TEST program (Tigecycline Evaluation and Surveillance Trial) showed a prevalence of 48% of MRSA in 2008 [7].

2. The molecular epidemiology of MRSA

Monitoring and stopping the intra- and inter-hospital distribution of MRSA clones require the use of efficient and accurate epidemiological typing systems that allow discrimination between unrelated isolates and recognition of isolates that descend from a common ancestor (i.e., that belong to the same clone). Currently, multiple phenotypic and genotypic typing methods have been developed to type MRSA. The choice of a typing method depends on the needs, the level of skills, the resources of the laboratory, and the type of question to be answered (short-term or long-term analysis) [8].

On the other hand, the molecular epidemiological study of MRSA aims to determine the clonal relationship that exists between several isolates of the same species. This information is very useful, especially when epidemic outbreaks caused by multi-resistant strains occur because it makes it possible to determine the number of circulating clones, evaluate the effectiveness of control measures aimed at preventing their spread, and differentiate between infection and reinfection [9]. Identification of MRSA clones is based on a combination of different typing methods, such as DNA hybridization with *mecA* and Tn554 probes, PFGE, RAPD, *SCCmec typing*, *spa typing*, and *MLST* [10].

3. International MRSA clones

At the present time, it has been shown that multiple clonal lineages of MRSA exist because of the successful horizontal transfer of *mecA* [11]. Six types of HA-MRSA hospital-acquired pandemic clones have been reported (Iberian, Brazilian, Hungarian, New York/Japan, Pediatric, and EMRSA-16), and they are scattered in different regions of the world [12]. The Iberian clone was the first one to be identified in 1989, in a massive outbreak of MRSA in a hospital in Barcelona, Spain [13]; but it seems to have already been present in Belgium and France at least since 1984 [14]. The Brazilian clone is widely distributed in Brazilian hospitals and has spread to neighboring countries in South America: Argentina, Uruguay and Chile and in Europe: Portugal, the Czech Republic, and Greece, where it displaced the main local clones [15]. The Hungarian clone has been widely disseminated in Hungarian hospitals since 1993 [16]. The New York/Japan clone was identified as the main clone in different regions in the United States of America [17], and in a hospital in Tokyo [18]. EMRSA-16 clone was found in the United Kingdom hospitals [19]. This clone has been widely spread in Greece, Mexico, and Canada [20]. The Pediatric clone was reported in Portugal in 1991 and since then, it has been found in Poland, France, the United Kingdom, the United States (EU), Argentina, and Colombia [21].

Reports of community-acquired methicillin-resistant *S. aureus* (CA-MRSA) infections in healthy people began to appear in the 1990s. In 2000, it was described that these types of strains were genetically different from bacteria isolated in hospital settings. Currently, CA-MRSA strain types possess more bacterial resistance genes, and more virulence factors, leading to more severe infections [22]. There are multiple clones of CA-MRSA worldwide, as well as a segregation of these clones based on the MLST technique. For example, USA300 (ST8), which predominates in the USA, USA400 (STI), USA1100 (ST30), and USA1000 (ST59), is clone notable for causing CA-MRSA infections. STI and ST30 are the cause of the main CA-MRSA infections in Australia and Oceania, while clone ST80 predominates in Europe [23].

The MRSA clones were once confined to hospitals for the last 20 years. MRSA infections have emerged in the community in people with no previous exposure to hospitals. Genotypically, CA-MRSA is a newer and more virulent strain, emerging in the late 1990s as leading the cause of skin and soft tissue infections in young healthy

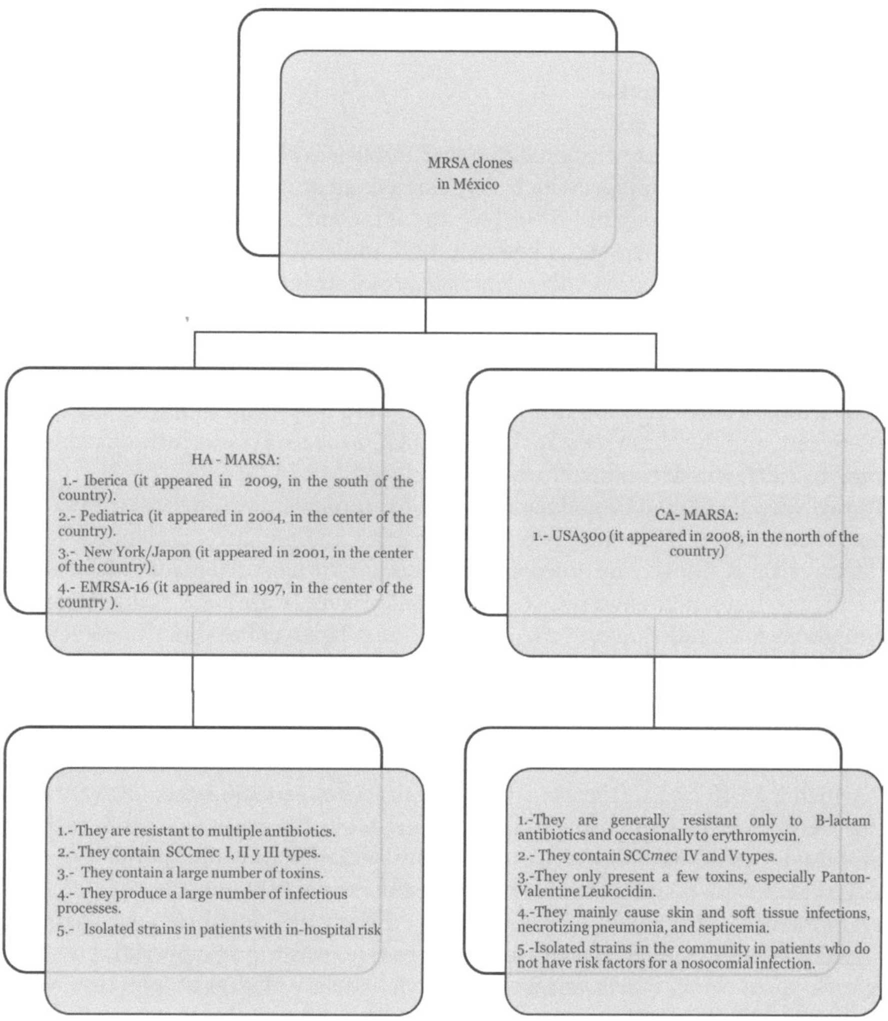

Figure 1.
Main differences between HA-MRSA and CA-MRSA strains detected in Mexico. (Modified by Bustos et al. [25]).

people. CA-MRSA strains typically carry *SCCmec types IV* or *V* and are generally susceptible to β-lactam antimicrobials. In addition, CA-MRSA carries Panton-Valentine Leukocidin (PVL), which is associated with increased pathogenicity. In relationship to HA-MRSA clones, they carry *SCCmec types I*, II, or III and do not have PVLs. HA-MRSA clones are associated with nosocomial infections, for example, endocarditis, urinary tract infections, and surgical infections, and are resistant to β-lactam antibiotics, especially aminoglycosides, macrolides, lincosamides, and fluoroquinolones. Although CA-MRSA has been predicted to replace HA-MRSA in hospitals, mathematical models predict the coexistence between the two strains given hospital-community interactions [24].

The molecular epidemiological study of MRSA clones has been insufficient in Mexico since there is not a systematized surveillance system, where the appearance or distribution of these clones is reported, monitored, and controlled. There have been few studies in Mexico over the years and they have randomly detected HA-MRSA and CA-MRSA clones in different states of the country, which have described their main phenotypic and genotypic characteristics, which are observed in **Figure 1**.

4. MRSA clones in Mexico

In Mexico, The Instituto Nacional de Salud Pública in México has been confirmed as a network of tertiary hospitals, which have carried out studies aimed at understanding the molecular epidemiology of MRSA [26] and it is coordinated by Dra. Velázquez-Meza and et al. Studies carried out between 1997 and 2003 at the Hospital de Pediatría del Centro Médico Nacional (CMN), Siglo XXI-IMSS (Mexican Institute of Social Security) in Mexico City, 659 strains of *S. aureus* were analyzed, with a variation in the prevalence of MRSA from 17 to 23% until 2001. It subsequently decreased drastically to a prevalence of 4% in 2002, which was due to nosocomial infection control measures. During this investigation, the presence of the clone EMRSA-16 (*SCCmec type IV*) was detected, and the clone New York/Japan (SCCmec *type II*) was introduced into the hospital in 2001, which completely displaced clone EMRSA-16 in 2002 [27].

At the Hospital Civil de Guadalajara, "Fray Antonio Alcalde" between 1999 and 2003, 839 strains of MRSA were isolated from adult and pediatric patients. A total of 216 MRSA strains showed antimicrobial resistance to β-lactams, macrolides, chloramphenicol, and imipenem, and sensitivity to gentamicin, rifampicin, trimethoprim-sulfamethoxazole, and vancomycin. The New York/Japan clone was also detected in the 216 MRSA strains studied, like the one found in the Hospital de Pediatría del CMN-Sigloi XXI [28]. The New York/Japan clone may have been transferred from the United States to Mexico.

At the Instituto de Cardiología "Dr. Ignacio Chavez" (ICh), located in Mexico City, which is a 246-bed tertiary teaching hospital between 2002 and 2009, 90 MRSA strains were collected from bronchial secretions, wound secretions, blood, catheter, pleural fluid, peritoneal fluid, and others, from pediatric and adult populations. MRSA isolates were resistant to amoxicillin, cefotaxime, cephalothin, cefazolin, chloramphenicol, imipenem, clindamycin, erythromycin, clarithromycin, penicillin, and oxacillin, while only 94.4% of isolates were also resistant to ciprofloxacin. The New York/Japan clone, which was isolated from a variety of sites of infection, was identified in 50% of MRSA isolates. The studies showed that the New York/Japan clone had *SCCmec type II*. EMRSA-16 was found in 2002 and it presented *SCCmec IV*, and this chromosomal cassette is related to CA-MRSA clones [29].

In the north of Mexico, an investigation was carried out to identify MRSA responsible for nosocomial infection in five medical centers in Monterrey, Nuevo León (NL) Mexico, between 2005 and 2009, and 190 strains of MRSA were isolated from five hospitals affiliated to the Mexican Institute of Social Security. This study clearly documented the high dissemination capacity and persistence of the New York/Japan clone in these centers [30].

At the Hospital San José Tec de Monterrey, Nuevo León, Mexico, the first five cases of a clone of community MRSA were described in 2008, and three of the patients were children. The first patient with a history of retinoblastoma in the left eye was diagnosed in November 2007, when he just started chemotherapy. In 2008, he returned to the hospital with a fever for 2 weeks of evolution. Blood cultures showed MRSA and vancomycin was started for 1 week. Two other children who were considered as healthy ones previously arrived at the hospital with abscesses and with a severe local reaction from where MRSA was isolated. After drainage, both were treated with clindamycin. Two other patients who were considered healthy adults previously had abscesses and because of it, they required hospitalization. The drainage of the lesions showed MRSA in the culture and the patients were treated with linezolid. All patients recovered. This study revealed that the pattern was similar to that observed for the CA-MRSA clone USA300 genotype [31].

On the other hand, at the Hospital Universitario Dr. José Eleuterio González, in Monterrey, between 2012 and 2013, a prophylactic protocol was carried out that consisted of applying a solution with chlorhexidine gluconate (CXG), throughout his body, with the aim of reducing nosocomial infections, where 158 strains of MRSA were collected. During these CXG washouts, antibiotic resistance significantly decreased for clindamycin, levofloxacin, and norfloxacin. During the pre-intervention period, 65.7% of the isolates were resistant to oxacillin, and in the post-intervention period, this percentage was reduced to 32.6%. This result indicates a significant reduction in the frequency of MRSA isolates as a result of the lavage with CXG. The presence of two clones descending from clone ST5-MRSA-II (New York/Japan) and clone ST8-MRSA-IV (USA300) was evidenced. The New York/Japan clone decreased significantly in the intervention period but recovered in the post-intervention period, while the USA300 clone was established under pressure from CXG [32].

Although in Monterrey, Mexico, the first clone of community origin of MRSA with a history in previously hospitalized patients was identified. In another study carried out in 2013 at the Universidad Autónoma Metropolitana-Xochimilco, in which healthy volunteers from schools and factories in Mexico City were recruited, to whom nasal or throat sampling was applied, a total of 131 strains of MRSA are obtained from 1039 strains of *S. aureus*. Considerable diversity in PFGE patterns in CA-MRSA isolates was observed in clonal analysis, allowing only a small number of clones to be detected: USA300 and USA100. This study provides the first description of CA-MRSA in healthy people in Mexico City, suggesting that community MRSA clones could replace hospital MRSA clones in the future [33].

At the Hospital de Oncología (INCAN), a tertiary care hospital in Mexico City in 2006 and later in 2010, the New York/Japan clone was isolated as the cause of an outbreak of nosocomial infections that arose from an index case [34, 35].

In relationship to MRSA clones in Veracruz, Veracruz, Mexico, at the Hospital Regional de Alta Especialidad in Veracruz (HRV) in 2010, the presence of two pandemic clones was identified, the New York/Japan clone (ST5-*SCCmec type II*) and the Iberian clone (ST247-*SCCmec type IA*). The IB1 clonal subtype was isolated from the emergency department in a patient with an ear infection, who stated that he had traveled to the USA, and on his return, he presented the infection, making it probable that the Iberian clone arrived from the USA to the HRV. The strains with IB2 and IB3 patterns were later isolated in two other patients from the same hospital medical service, which reveals the introduction of this clone from an external service to a critical area of the HRV [36]. Although the New York/Japan clone has been previously identified in other hospitals in Mexico [12, 13, 31], this clearly demonstrates its great capacity for geographical expansion, multi-resistance, and virulence. The importance of this finding lies in the fact that the first strain of MRSA resistant to vancomycin with a minimum inhibitory concentration (MIC) of 1024 μg/ml belongs to the New York/Japan lineage [37, 38].

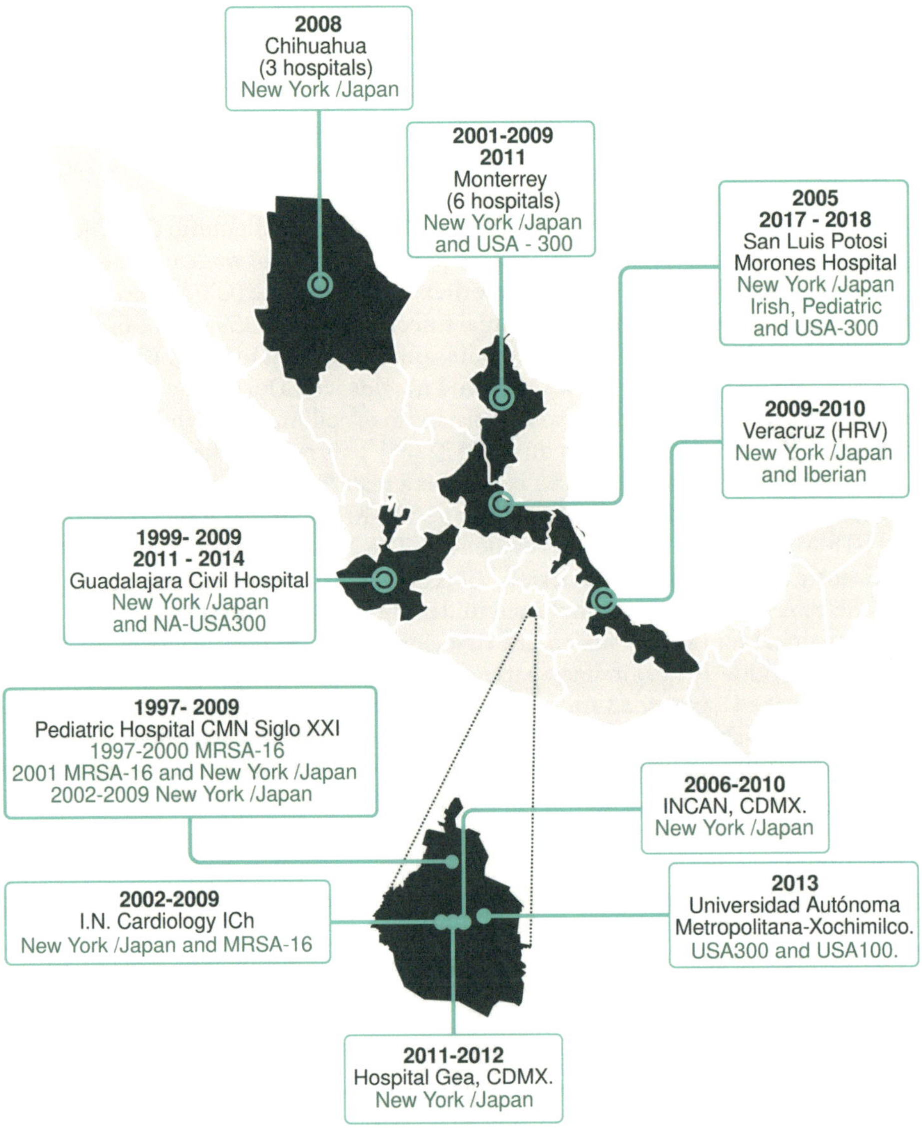

Figure 2.
Distribution of MRSA clones in Mexico.

At the Hospital General "Dr. Manuel Gea González," located in the southern zone of Mexico City, from 2011 to 2012, 109 strains of MRSA were isolated from wound secretions, soft tissues, blood cultures, cerebrospinal fluid, pleural fluid, bone, etc., of hospitalized patients. The most prevalent infection was ventilator-associated pneumonia. The isolated strains were characterized by resistance to β-lactams. A single predominant clone named New York/Japan (NY) was identified [39].

A prospective observational cohort study was carried out and 24 hospitals in Latin America participated from 2011 to 2014 and collected 1346 strains of *S. aureus*. The Hospital Civil de Guadalajara, Fray Antonio Alcalde de Guadalajara, Mexico, participated, and 18% of the MRSA isolates in this hospital showed the typical pattern of USA300, suggesting that this strain is likely circulating in Mexico [40].

In a cross-sectional study carried out at the Hospital Central Dr. Ignacio Morones Prieto, in San Luis Potosí, Mexico, from 2017 to 2018, a total of 191 isolates of *S. aureus* were obtained from different patients in all wards of the hospital, in the pediatric and adult population, coming from the emergency services, surgery, intensive care unit, internal medicine, gynecology, burn unit, and outpatient service. Clinical samples were obtained from skin and soft tissue infections, respiratory tract, blood, bones and joints, and the cerebrospinal fluid. A total of 77% of the strains were considered as coming to the hospital and 23% were classified as community ones. The most frequent *S. aureus* infections were those that affected the skin, soft tissues, and bacteremia. Instead, the type of infection more frequent cause by isolates of MRSA was the infection of the surgical site. The presence of clones ST5-MRSA-II-t895 (clone New York/Japan) and ST1011-MRSA-II-t9364 (clone New York/Japan) was evidenced by the PFGE technique. In addition to the clone mentioned above, the presence of endemic clones of MRSA was evidenced, such as USA300, Irish and Pediatric, these being the ones with the highest prevalence [41].

As seen in previous studies in Mexico, the predominant clone is the New York/Japan [42], which has the ability to spread, cause outbreaks and replace existing clones [43], and this is due, among other things, to its great virulence, since it presents staphylococcal enterotoxins and it also possesses the toxic shock syndrome toxin 1, which enables it to cause a wide variety of clinical syndromes, including toxic shock syndrome and suppurative infections [44]. In addition to this, it is resistant to β-lactams and a wide range of antibiotics [15].

The epidemiological study of MRSA clones acquired in hospitals is an area of little study, which does not allow knowing exactly the behavior or evolution of MRSA pandemic clones, as shown in the following **Figure 2**, which compiles the reported clones in Mexico.

5. Conclusions

It is necessary to promote and encourage the molecular epidemiological surveillance of HA-MRSA and CA-MRSA clones, to prevent and control this pathogen, which causes outbreaks and high mortality rates in Mexico, due to hospital or community infections. Attention shoulder be paid to the detection, surveillance, and control of CA-MRSA due to the increase in the non-hospitalized population, which could displace HA-MRSA and become a health problem.

The molecular epidemiological surveillance of MRSA clones is essential knowledge for its prevention, control, and possible eradication. This type of research allows the nosocomial infection control committees of each institution to be informed. This in sum would help to strengthen measures, such as the restriction of prescription of broad-spectrum antibiotics, daily supervision of cultures and results, monthly reports of infections, training aimed at health workers in general, and strengthening of medical practices.

In Mexico, the predominant clone is New York/Japan, which has the ability to spread, cause outbreaks and replace existing clones, this is due, among other things, to its great virulence and antimicrobial multi-resistance. The importance of this clone lies in the fact that the first strain of MRSA resistant to vancomycin belongs to the New York/Japan lineage. Vancomycin is considered one of the latest therapeutic alternatives against infections caused by MRSA and other gram-positive microorganisms.

Author details

Miguel Ángel Ortíz Gil* and Monica Irasu Cardona Alvarado
Department of Medical Science, Division of Health Sciences, Leon Campus, University of Guanajuato, Leon, México

*Address all correspondence to: maortiz@ugto.mx

References

[1] Selvey LA, Whitby M, Johnson B. Nosocomial methicillin-resistant Staphylococcus aureus bacteremia: Is it any worse than nosocomial methicillin-sensitive Staphylococcus aureus bacteremia? Infection Control and Hospital Epidemiology. 2000;**21**(10): 645-648. DOI: 10.1086/501707

[2] Dinges MM, Orwin PM, Schlievert PM. Exotoxins of Staphylococcus aureus. Clinical Microbiology Reviews. 2000;**13**(1):16-34. DOI: 10.1128/cmr.13.1.16

[3] Milheiriço C, Oliveira DC, de Lencastre H. Update to the multiplex PCR strategy for assignment of mec element types in Staphylococcus aureus. Antimicrobial Agents and Chemotherapy. 2007;**51**(9):3374-3377. DOI: 10.1128/AAC.00275-07

[4] Chambers HF. Methicillin resistance in staphylococci: Molecular and biochemical basis and clinical implications. Clinical Microbiology Reviews. 1997;**10**(4):781-791. DOI: 10.1128/CMR.10.4.781

[5] Chambers HF. Methicillin-resistant staphylococci. Clinical Microbiology Reviews. 1988;**1**(2):173-186. DOI: 10.1128/CMR.1.2.173

[6] López IKR, Hernández JBBD, Rosas DOP, Camacho MV, Ruiz ÉMF, Novales MGM. Bacterial resistance in isolates from patients with nosocomial infections. Enfermedades Infecciosas y Microbiología. 2007;**27**(1):15-21

[7] Guzmán BM, Mejía C, Isturiz R, Alvarez C, Bavestrello L, Gotuzzo E, et al. Epidemiology of methicillin-resistant Staphylococcus aureus (MRSA) in Latin America. International Journal of Antimicrobial Agents. 2009;**34**:304-308

[8] Struelens MJ. Consensus guidelines for appropriate use and evaluation of microbial epidemiologic typing systems. Clinical Microbiology and Infection. 1996;**2**(1):2-11. DOI: 10.1111/j.1469-0691.1996.tb00193.x

[9] Fernández-Cuenca F. Aplicaciones de las técnicas de PCR a la epidemiología molecular de las enfermedades infecciosas. Enfermedades Infecciosas y Microbiología Clínica. 2004;**22**(6): 355-360. DOI: 10.1157/13063748

[10] Castellano GM, Perozo MA, Vivas VR, Ginestre PM, Rincón VG. Tipificación molecular y fenotípica de Staphylococcus aureus resistentes a meticilina (SAMR) en un hospital universitario. Revista Chilena de Infectología. 2009;**26**:39-48

[11] Fluit AC, Schmitz FJ. MRSA: Current Perspectives. EEUU: Edit. Horizon Scientific Press; 2003

[12] Lencastre H, Oliveira D, Tomasz A. Antibiotic resistant Staphylococcus aureus: A paradigm of adaptive power. Current Opinion in Microbiology. 2007;**10**:428-435

[13] Oliveira DC, Tomasz A, De Lencastre H. The evolution of pandemic clones of methicillin-resistant Staphylococcus aureus: Identication of two ancestral genetic backgrounds and the associated mec elements. Microbial Drug Resistance. 2001;**7**:349-361

[14] Deplano A, Witte W, van Leeuwen WJ, Brun Y, Struelens MJ. Clonal dissemination of epidemic methicillin-resistant Staphylococcus

aureus in Belgium and neighboring countries. Clinical Microbiology and Infection. 2000;**6**(5):239-245. DOI: 10.1046/j.1469-0691.2000.00064.x

[15] Teixeira LA, Resende CA, Ormonde LR, Rosenbaum R, Figueiredo AM, de Lencastre H, et al. Geographic spread of epidemic multiresistant Staphylococcus aureus clone in Brazil. Journal of Clinical Microbiology. 1995;**33**(9):2400-2404. DOI: 10.1128/jcm.33.9.2400-2404.1995

[16] Aires de Sousa M, Crisóstomo MI, Sanches IS, Wu JS, Fuzhong J, Tomasz A, et al. Frequent recovery of a single clonal type of multidrug-resistant Staphylococcus aureus from patients in two hospitals in Taiwan and China. Journal of Clinical Microbiology. 2003;**41**(1):159-163. DOI: 10.1128/JCM.41.1.159-163.2003

[17] Simor AE, Ofner-Agostini M, Bryce E, Mcgeer A, Paton S, Mulvey MR. Laboratory characterization of methicillin resistant Staphylococcus aureus in Canadian hospitals: Results of 5 years of National Surveillance, 1995-1999. The Journal of Infectious Diseases. 2002;**186**:652-660

[18] Aires de Sousa M, de Lencastre H, Santos Sanches I, Kikuchi K, Totsuka K, Tomasz A. Similarity of antibiotic resistance patterns and molecular typing properties of methicillin-resistant Staphylococcus aureus isolates widely spread in hospitals in new York City and in a hospital in Tokyo, Japan. Microbial Drug Resistance. 2000 Autumn;**6**(3):253-258. DOI: 10.1089/mdr.2000.6.253

[19] Moore PC, Lindsay JA. Molecular characterization of the dominant UK methicillin-resistant Staphylococcus aureus strains, EMRSA-15 and EMRSA-16. Journal of Medical Microbiology. 2002;**51**:516-521

[20] Murchan S, Kaufmann ME, Deplano A, de Ryck R, Struelens M, Zinn CE, et al. Harmonization of pulsed field gel electrophoresis for epidemiological typing of methicillin-resistant Staphylococcus aureus by consensus in 10 European centers and its use to plot the spread of related strains. Journal of Clinical Microbiology. 2003;**41**:1574-1585

[21] Aires de Sousa M, de Lencastre H. Bridges from hospitals to the laboratory: Genetic portraits of methicillin-resistant Staphylococcus aureus clones. FEMS Immunology and Medical Microbiology. 2004;**40**(2):101-111. DOI: 10.1016/s0928-8244(03)00370-5

[22] Castañeda-Méndez PF. Frecuencia de infecciones por S. aureus en pacientes hospitalizados en un hospital privado de tercer nivel de la Ciudad de México. Revista Médica MD. 2018;**9**:317-321

[23] García EC, González RG, Schettino PMS. Staphylococcus aureus asociado a la comunidad. Revista Mexicana de Patología Clínica y Medicina de Laboratorio. 2015;**62**:100-111

[24] Kateete DP et al. CA-MRSA and HA-MRSA coexist in community and hospital settings in Uganda. Antimicrobial Resistance & Infection Control. 2019;**8**(1):1-9

[25] Bustos J, Hamdan A, Gutiérrez M. Staphylococcus aureus: la reemergencia de un patógeno en la comunidad. Revista Biomedica. 2006;**17**(4):287-305

[26] Aires De Sousa M, Miragaia M, Sanches IS, Avila S, Adamson I, Casagrande ST, et al. Three-year assessment of methicillin-resistant Staphylococcus aureus clones in

Latin America from 1996 to 1998. Journal of Clinical Microbiology. 2001;**39**(6):2197-2205. DOI: 10.1128/JCM.39.6.2197-2205.2001

[27] Velazquez-Meza ME, Aires de Sousa M, Echaniz-Aviles G, Solórzano-Santos F, Miranda-Novales G, Silva-Sanchez J, et al. Surveillance of methicillin-resistant Staphylococcus aureus in a pediatric hospital in Mexico City during a 7-year period (1997 to 2003): Clonal evolution and impact of infection control. Journal of Clinical Microbiology. 2004;**42**(8):3877-3880. DOI: 10.1128/JCM.42.8.3877-3880.2004

[28] Echániz-Aviles G, Velázquez-Meza ME, Aires-de-Sousa M, Morfín-Otero R, Rodríguez-Noriega E, Carnalla-Barajas N, et al. Molecular characterisation of a dominant methicillin-resistant Staphylococcus aureus (MRSA) clone in a Mexican hospital (1999-2003). Clinical Microbiology and Infection. 2006;**12**(1):22-28. DOI: 10.1111/j.1469-0691.2005.01283.x

[29] Elena V-MM et al. Pulsed field gel electrophoresis in molecular typing and epidemiological detection of methicillin resistant Staphylococcus aureus (MRSA). Gel Electrophoresis–Advanced Techniques. 2012;**10**:179

[30] Velazquez-Meza ME, Hernández-Salgado M, Contreras-Cordero JF, Pérez-Cortes P, Villarreal-Treviño L. Surveillance of methicillin-resistant staphylococcus aureus causing nosocomial infections in five medical centers of Monterrey, Nuevo León, México from 2005-2009. Archives of Medical Research. 2013;**44**(7):570-574. DOI: 10.1016/j.arcmed.2013.09.001

[31] Velazquez-Meza ME, Ayala-Gaytán J, Carnalla-Barajas MN, Soto-Noguerón A, Guajardo-Lara CE, Echaniz-Aviles G. First report of community-associated methicillin-resistant Staphylococcus aureus (USA300) in Mexico. Journal of Clinical Microbiology. 2011;**49**(8):3099-3100. DOI: 10.1128/JCM.00533-11

[32] Velázquez-Meza ME, Mendoza-Olazarán S, Echániz-Aviles G, Camacho-Ortiz A, Martínez-Reséndez MF, Valero-Moreno V, et al. Chlorhexidine whole-body washing of patients reduces methicillin-resistant Staphylococcus aureus and has a direct effect on the distribution of the ST5-MRSA-II (New York/Japan) clone. Journal of Medical Microbiology. 2017;**66**(6):721-728. DOI: 10.1099/jmm.0.000487

[33] Hamdan-Partida A, Sainz-Espuñes T, Bustos-Martínez J. Isolation of community-acquired methicillin-resistant Staphylococcus aureus in healthy carriers in a Mexican community. International Journal of Infectious Diseases. 2014;**18**:22-26. DOI: 10.1016/j.ijid.2013.08.010

[34] Cornejo-Juárez P, Velásquez-Acosta C, Díaz-González A, Volkow-Fernández P. Tendencia del perfil de sensibilidad antimicrobiana de los aislamientos de sangre en un hospital oncológico (1998-2003). Salud Pública de México. 2005;**47**(4):288-293. DOI: 10.1590/s0036-36342005000400006

[35] Cornejo-Juárez P, Volkow-Fernández P, Sifuentes-Osornio J, Echániz-Aviles G, Díaz-Gonzalez A, Velázquez-Acosta C, et al. Tracing the source of an outbreak of methicillin-resistant Staphylococcus aureus in a tertiary-care oncology hospital by epidemiology and molecular methods. Microbial Drug Resistance. 2010;**16**(3):203-208. DOI: 10.1089/mdr.2010.0048

[36] Ortíz-Gil MÁ, Velazquez-Meza ME, Echániz-Aviles G, Mora-Domínguez JP,

Carnalla-Barajas MN, Mendiola Del Moral EL. Tracking methicillin-resistant Staphylococcus aureus clones in a hospital in southern Mexico. Salud Pública de México. 2020;**62**(2):186-191. DOI: 10.21149/10786

[37] McDougal LK, Steward CD, Killgore GE, Chaitram JM, McAllister SK, Tenover FC. Pulsed-field gel electrophoresis typing of oxacillin-resistant Staphylococcus aureus isolates from the United States: Establishing a national database. Journal of Clinical Microbiology. 2003;**41**(11):5113-5120. DOI: 10.1128/JCM.41.11.5113-5120.2003

[38] Weigel LM, Clewell DB, Gill SR, Clark NC, McDougal LK, Flannagan SE, et al. Genetic analysis of a high-level vancomycin-resistant isolate of Staphylococcus aureus. Science. 2003;**302**(5650):1569-1571. DOI: 10.1126/science.1090956

[39] Gasca S, De H, Meza V, Avilés E, Castro V, Moreno F. Caracterización molecular de cepas de S. aureus meticilino resistentes (MRSA) aisladas en pacientes del Hospital General "Dr. Manuel Gea González". [Tesis doctoral]. Instituto de Salud Pública: Cuernavaca, Morelos; 2013. https://catalogoinsp.mx/files/tes/053411.pdf

[40] Arias CA, Reyes J, Carvajal LP, Rincon S, Diaz L, Panesso D, et al. A prospective cohort multicenter study of molecular epidemiology and phylogenomics of Staphylococcus aureus bacteremia in nine Latin American countries. Antimicrobial Agents and Chemotherapy. 2017;**61**(10):e00816-17. DOI: 10.1128/aac.00816-17

[41] Negrete-González C, Turrubiartes-Martínez E, Galicia-Cruz OG, Noyola DE, Martínez-Aguilar G, Pérez-González LF, et al. High prevalence of t895 and t9364 spa types of methicillin-resistant Staphylococcus aureus in a tertiary-care hospital in Mexico: Different lineages of clonal complex 5. BMC Microbiology. 2020;**20**(1):213. DOI: 10.1186/s12866-020-01881-w

[42] Coombs GW, Van Gessel H, Pearson JC, Godsell M-R, O'Brien FG, Christiansen KJ. Controlling a multicenter outbreak involving the New York/Japan methicillin-resistant Staphylococcus aureus clone. Infection Control and Hospital Epidemiology. 2007;**28**(7):845-852. DOI: 10.1086/518726

[43] Orii KO, Iwao Y, Higuchi W, Takano T, Yamamoto T. Molecular characterization of methicillin-resistant Staphylococcus aureus from a fatal case of necrotizing fasciitis in an extremely low-birth-weight infant. Clinical Microbiology and Infection. 2010;**16**(3):289-292. DOI: 10.1111/j.1469-0691.2009.02806.x

[44] Durand G, Bes M, Meugnier H, Enright MC, Forey F, Liassine N, et al. Detection of new methicillin-resistant Staphylococcus aureus clones containing the toxic shock syndrome toxin 1 gene responsible for hospital- and community-acquired infections in France. Journal of Clinical Microbiology. 2006;**44**(3):847-853

Chapter 4

Main Factors of *Staphylococcus aureus* Associated with the Interaction to the Cells for Their Colonization and Persistence

Samuel González-García, Aída Hamdan-Partida, Juan José Valdez-Alarcón, Anaid Bustos-Hamdan and Jaime Bustos-Martínez

Abstract

Staphylococcus aureus is a microorganism that can colonize the nose, pharynx, and other regions of the body. It has also been observed that it can cause persistence. Successful colonization of *S. aureus* depends in the factors that favor the interaction of the bacteria with host cells. The bacterial determinants of *S. aureus* that have the capacity to adhere to human tissues involve adhesion factors such as teichoic acids and cell-wall-anchored proteins (CWA) such as ClfA, IcaA, SdrC, FnBPA, among others. The colonization and persistence process first involve adhesion to the tissue, followed by its reproduction and the possible formation of a biofilm. This review will describe the main virulence factors that allow bacterial adhesion and biofilm formation, including the accessory gene regulator genes (*agr*), related to colonization and persistence of *S. aureus*.

Keywords: *S. aureus*, colonization, persistence, adhesins, biofilm, virulence factors, regulation, *agr*

1. Introduction

Staphylococcus aureus is a versatile pathogen that can cause infections in several mammal species including human. This is possible because several genetic variants have been associated with the host and the type of infection [1]. *S. aureus* can form a normal part of the human microbiota or act as an opportunistic pathogenic bacterium that produces a wide range of diseases that can be acquired in the hospital or in the community [2].

Several studies of colonization of *S. aureus* in the nose show that it can persist, following three patterns of carriers in the population. Around 20% of people are persistent carriers, around 30% are intermittent carriers, and non-carriers are on average 50% [3]. It has been reported that persistent carriers usually present a single strain over time, shed the bacteria in the environment, and they can be infected more than intermittent carriers and non-carriers. Intermittent carriers may have different strains over time and less colonization [4].

In the adults *S. aureus* can be found apart from the nose at other sites in the body: pharynx (4–64%), abdomen (15%), armpits (8%), intestines (17–31%), perineum (22%), and vagina (5%) [5–7].

Bacterial adhesion to the skin or mucous membranes is usually the initial and fundamental step in colonization and persistence, with the subsequent possibility of producing infections and pathological processes in the host. By attaching, bacteria can also bypass the innate response, allowing access to nutrients, colonization, and possibly subsequent persistence, which is favored by biofilm formation, toxin production, cell invasion, and evasion mechanisms of the immune response [8].

2. Colonization factors of *S. aureus*

Colonization with *S. aureus* requires direct human contact or contact with contaminated fomites. But this does not guarantee colonization, and some people remain as non-carriers [9]. Once colonizing, permanence is an important trail in persistent infections. Therefore, it is required to study the factors involved in colonization and persistence.

2.1 Initial *S. aureus* interaction

Colonization begins by the interaction of the bacteria with the cells of the host. *S. aureus* has many adhesins that allow it to first adhere to the human cell, multiply, and even persist in the tissue. Next, several components of the bacterium that intervene in the interaction with the host are reviewed.

2.1.1 Wall teichoic acids (WTA)

Reversible binding of *S. aureus* to host cells is through wall teichoic acids (WTAs) and/or receptor-mediated protein interactions [10]. The surface of *S. aureus* is composed of polysaccharides, such as capsular polysaccharides (PC) and also by WTA. Two types of acids have been described: lipoteichoic acids (LTA), which are found in the cytoplasmic membrane, and teichoic acids (WTAs), which are bound to peptidoglycan in the cell wall [11, 12]. WTAs are found on the surface of the cell wall, which are polyanionic cell wall glycopolymers (CWGs). They are made up of approximately 40 repeat units of ribitolphosphate linked with D-alanine and N-acetylglucosamine, which are covalently linked to peptidoglycan [13, 14].

WTAs have been shown to participate in the adhesion and colonization of staphylococci [14, 15], also participate in cell division, as well as in the formation of biofilms, an elevated expression increases the virulence of *S. aureus* [16]. It has also been seen that the D-alanine residues of the WTA participate in resistance against antimicrobial peptides (defensins or cathelicidins), in addition to participating in the resistance of some antibiotics such as teicoplanin or vancomycin [11, 17]. The biosynthesis of these biopolymers in *S. aureus* is mediated by N-acetylglucosaminyltransferase (Tar) enzymes [18].

Weidenmaier et al. [19], using a *S. aureus* model for nasal colonization in cotton rats, found that the proteinaceous adhesins of the bacterium act mainly during the later stages of colonization, while the non-proteinaceous WTA-type adhesin acts in the early stages. This is due to the high expression of the WTA *tagO* and *tarK* genes during the first and last stages of colonization, while the expression of adhesin proteins such as clumping factor B (ClfB) increases in the early stages and decreases in the later stages of colonization [14, 20–22]. Therefore, WTA is not required for the *in vitro* growth of *S. aureus*; however, it is required for establishing infection in animals [18].

The action of WTA in the initial interaction of *S. aureus* to a surface is through non-covalent surface charge interactions (WTA is a polyanionic molecule), with various associated polymeric proteins in the cell membrane (recently its interaction with the Scavenger receptor SREC-1) having been demonstrated, which allows its adhesion to the structural molecules of the cell matrix such as fibronectin, fibrinogen, collagen, etc. [23, 24].

2.1.2 S. aureus cell wall-anchored (CWA) proteins

S. aureus has been shown to produce some 25 different cell-wall-anchored (CWA) proteins, linked to peptidoglycan via transpeptidases. These CWA may function in adhesion, biofilm formation, invasion, and evasion of host immune responses [25].

Five groups have been proposed to classify *S. aureus* CWA proteins (**Table 1**). Where there are many microbial surface components recognizing adhesive matrix molecules (MSCRAMM), including fibronectin-binding proteins (FnBPA and FnBPB), proteins of the Serine-Aspartate repeat family (SdrC, SdrD, and SdrE), clumping factors (ClfA and ClfB), Protein A (Spa), iron-regulated surface determinants (IsdA, IsdB, IsdC, and IsdH), plasmin-responsive protein (Pls), *S. aureus* surface protein G (SasG), and bone sialoprotein-binding protein (Bbp). All of these proteins participate in the initial interaction with the host cell through cell adhesion and/or biofilm formation [26].

2.1.2.1 Microbial surface components recognizing adhesive matrix molecules (MSCRAMM) used to attach to cells

S. aureus reversibly or irreversibly binds to the cell surface via MSCRAMM proteins [25, 27]. During infection, these proteins allow bacteria to bind to host receptors. These proteins are made up of three parts: a binding domain, a domain that spans the entire cell wall, and a third part on the bacterial surface that serves for non-covalent binding of MSCRAMM proteins to the host cell [25, 26].

The main binding factors of *S. aureus* (**Table 1**) are reviewed below.

2.1.2.1.1 Clumping factor B (ClfB)

S. aureus binds to nostrils during colonization via clumping factor B (ClfB) by highly affine binding to the cornified cell envelope, mainly due to the fibrinogen binding mechanism, which is an important step in colonization by *S. aureus* [28, 29], as well as *in vitro* biofilm formation [30]. Therefore, the union of ClfB with fibrinogen promotes nasal colonization. ClfB expression occurs mainly in the early phase of bacterial exponential growth and is de-expressed in the late growth phase and stationary phase [31]. Most strains of *S. aureus* have the *clfB* gene [21, 32, 33]. The ClfB protein exhibits sequence variations depending on *S. aureus* clonal complexes, but protein variants have about 94% amino acid identity with each other [34].

Protein group	Ligand	Function
1. MSCRAMM		
Clumping factor A (ClfA)	Fibrinogen Complement factor I	Fibrinogen binding, evades immune response by binding to soluble fibrinogen Evasion of the immune response; C3b degradation
Clumping factor B (ClfB)	Fibrinogen, loricrin, keratin 10; DLL	Adherence to desquamated epithelial cells. Participates in nasal colonization
Protein C with Serine-aspartate repeats (SdrC)	B-neurexin; DLL Desquamated epithelial cells	Unknown Possible nasal colonization
Protein D with Serine-aspartate repeats (SdrD)	Desquamated epithelial cells	Possible nasal colonization
Serine-aspartate repeat-containing Protein E (SdrE)	Complement factor H	Evasion of the immune response; C3b degradation
Bone sialoprotein-binding protein (SdrE isoform)	Fibrinogen; DLL	Adhesion to the extracellular matrix (ECM)
Fibronectin binding proteins A (FnBPA) and B (FnBPB)	Fibrinogen and elastin, DLL. FnBPA domain A also binds fibronectin, but not by DLL Fibronectin	Adhesion to ECM Adhesion to ECM; invasion
Collagen adhesin (Cna)	Collagen	Adhesion to collagen-rich tissues
2. NEAT (near iron transporter) motif family		
Iron-regulated surface protein A (IsdA)	Heme, fibronectin, fibrinogen, loricrin, cytokeratin 10, Unknown ligand (NEAT motif region of C-terminal domain)	Heme absorption and iron acquisition; adhesion to desquamated epithelial cells; lactoferrin resistance Resistance to antimicrobial peptides and bactericidal lipids; neutrophil infection
Iron-regulated surface protein B (IsdB)	Hemoglobin, Heme β3 integrins	Heme absorption and iron acquisition Invasion of non-phagocytic cells
Iron-regulated surface protein H (IsdH)	Heme, hemoglobin Unknown ligand (NEAT motif region of the N-terminal domain	Heme absorption and iron acquisition Accelerated degradation of C3b
3. Three helix packaging		
Protein A	IgG Fc, IgM Fab subclass VH3, TNFR1 von Willebrand factor Unknown ligand (Xr region)	Inhibition of phagocytosis; B cell superantigen; inflammation Endovascular infection; endocarditis Inflammation
4. G5-E repeat family		
S. aureus surface protein G (SasG) and plasmin-sensitive surface protein (Pls) (a homolog of SasG in MRSA)	Unknown ligand (A domain) Unknown ligand (G5-E repeats)	Adhesion of desquamated epithelial cells Biofilm formation
5. Structurally uncharacterized proteins		

Protein group	Ligand	Function
Adenosine synthase A (AdsA)	Non-link-mediated function	Survival in neutrophils by inhibiting oxidative processes
S. aureus surface protein X (SasX)	Unknown ligand	Biofilm formation, cell aggregation, and squamous cell adhesion
Serine-rich adhesin for platelets (SraP)	Salivary agglutinin gp340 and an unidentified ligand on platelets	Endocarditis; and endovascular infection
S. aureus surface protein C (SasC)	Unknown ligand	Induces the primary attachment of cells and their accumulation in the formation of biofilms
SasB, SasF, SasF, SasJ, SasK and SasL	Unknown ligands	Possible LPXTG proteins. Unknown structure or function
Biofilm-associated protein (Bap)	gp96	It stimulates the formation of biofilms and aggregation on the surfaces of epithelial cells, prevents the invasion of epithelial cells of the mammary glands. It is only found in bovine strains.

ECM: extracellular matrix; DLL: dock, lock and latch. The shaded rows belong to the main ligands of S. aureus to the host (modified from Foster et al. [25]).

Table 1.
Main cell-wall-anchored (CWA) proteins of Staphylococcus aureus.

ClfB also binds to cytokeratin 10, in addition to binding fibrinogen, cytokeratin 10 is one of the main components of the interior of squamous cells. ClfB also binds loricrin, one of the most abundant protein in the cornified envelope of squamous cells, and is key in the colonization of *S. aureus* in the nose and human skin [28, 29, 31, 34, 35]. Initially, it was found that the ClfB protein binds to fibrinogen, it can undergo the proteolytic action of the *S. aureus* metalloprotease aureolysin [36]. ClfB protein in digested form cannot bind fibrinogen, but can bind cytokeratin 10 with good affinity. At the ligand level, ClfB interacts with the amino acid sequence Y[GS]nY found in the carboxyl-terminal of cytokeratin 10 [37].

The ClfB binding is carried out using the so-called dock, lock, and latch (DLL) mechanism, where a short peptide of cytokeratin 10 or loricrin binds the N2 and N3 domains of the ClfB protein [38, 39].

2.1.2.1.2 Serine-aspartate repeats (SdrC and SdrD) proteins

Within the MSCRAMM is the subfamily of serine-aspartate repeat (Sdr) proteins, which have an R region that presents repeats of the serine-aspartate dipeptide and is located in the sdr locus [38, 40]. In *S. aureus*, three members of Sdr are known, and they are SdrC, SdrD, and SdrE, which share a conserved structure [38].

Askarian et al. [41] reported that SdrD is required for survival of *S. aureus* within the host, giving it the ability to evade some processes of the innate immune response, particularly by inactivating the complement system through the lectin pathway. On the other hand, SdrE functions in the recognition of complement binding protein C4b.(C4BP) [42, 43]. On the other hand, SdrC is important for the formation of bacterial biofilms [44]. SdrC can also bind specifically and with high affinity to β-neurexin [45]. *S. aureus* has at least two of the sdr genes, with the sdrC gene always being found, the other two may or may not be in the *S. aureus* genome [40]. Strains that possess only the sdrC gene are less likely to cause bone infections, because it is related to one of the SdrE variants that has been identified as a bone sialoprotein-binding protein [46]. SdrD is crucial for abscess formation and can interact with desmoglein (desmosomal protein that maintains the structure of the epidermis through its adhesive function) [41, 47, 48].

2.1.2.2 Iron-regulated surface proteins (Isd)

Iron-regulated surface proteins (Isd) are responsible for transporting the heme group, the system is made up of nine proteins (IsdA-IsdI) and are activated if the bacterium has iron-limited conditions [21, 49, 50]. The heme group binds to a membrane, and from there it passes to the cytoplasm, once at this site, the heme oxygenases release the iron atoms [25]. *S. aureus* requires these hemoproteins for growth and virulence [51, 52].

Isd proteins present domains of the nearby iron transporter (NEAr iron Transporter, NEAT), which participate in the capture of the heme group of hemoglobin, favoring the development of bacteria in the host in places where there is low iron concentration. Isd proteins have NEAT domains, which vary according to the type of Isd, since IsdA only has one, IsdB has two, and IsdH has three, with which it can bind to the heme group, IsdA also has a hydrophilic end C-terminal, which is responsible for decreasing the hydrophobicity of the cell surface, making the bacteria resistant to lipid bactericides and other antimicrobial peptides [25].

Isd proteins are important during bacterial pathogenesis. IsdA can bind to various host proteins in addition to the heme group (fibrinogen, fibronectin, cytokeratin 10, etc.), promoting adherence to cell lines and tissues, and acts together with IsdB to provide resistance to neutrophil killing [53].

2.1.2.3 S. aureus surface proteins (SasG and SasX)

There is a broad association between *S. aureus* surface protein G (SasG) and accumulation-associated protein (Aap), the latter being required by *Staphylococcus epidermidis* for biofilm formation and promoting intercellular adhesion [54, 55].

SasG binds covalently to the cell wall via homophilic protein-protein interactions through Zn^{2+}-dependent cleaved SasG B domains, resulting in cell-cell adhesion. However, the host cell binding ligand is still unknown [56–59].

S. aureus colonizes the nasal epithelium mainly due to ClfB and IsdA proteins, which allow adhesion to desquamated epithelial cells [25]. However, adhesion to epithelial cells is also promoted by SasG and may contribute to colonization [60]. In addition, overexpression of the *sasG* gene can inhibit clumping proteins (ClfA and ClfB) to increase biofilm formation [61, 62].

SasX protein, another CWA protein, seems to have been important in the epidemics caused by MRSA in hospitals on the Asian continent [63]. The *sasX* gene is known to be encoded by a bacteriophage that is in lysogenic form [34], SasX protein increases the formation of biofilms, by increasing cell aggregation it leads to a decrease in phagocytosis of neutrophils [63, 64] and adhesion to desquamated cells [25]. Therefore, the *sasX* gene not only encodes a colonization factor but also helps virulence of *S. aureus* by evading immune response [65]. SasX has also been associated with disease severity in skin and lung infections [63].

2.1.3 Adhesins regulation

The regulation of the virulence factors of *S. aureus* is carried out by a system that integrates signals derived from the host and the environment in a coordinated manner. Two-Component Systems (TCSs) are processes that identify environmental changes and produce regulation. Generally, membrane-associated histidine kinase is activated by an external signal, this induces its autophosphorylation and then phosphorylates a regulatory protein. This phosphorylated protein can bind to a specific DNA sequence, causing altered expression of the target gene. The majority of *S. aureus* strains have 16 different TCSs [66], the WalR/WalS system involved in regulating cell wall metabolism is essential, and some of the other 15 may be inactivated in various strains [67, 68]. Other TCSs such as arlRS, agrAC, and saeRS are implicated in *S. aureus* virulence by regulating many secreted proteins that affect the host [69].

2.1.3.1 Accessory gene regulator (Agr) system

Among the most studied regulatory systems is the accessory gene regulator (Agr), which is responsible for encoding a *quorum sensing* system that serves as the master regulator of virulence [69].

The Agr system detects a signal given by an autoinducer peptide (AIP), composed of 7–9 amino acids. There are four different alleles for the *agr* locus, each strain presenting only one of them. All four known *S. aureus* AIPs contain a cysteine residue that forms a cyclic thiolactone ring with the carboxylate at the C-terminal end of the peptide, which seems to be essential for its function [70]. Once the peptide AIP reaches the critical concentration or depletion of glucose in the extracellular medium, the system is activated in the quorum cells of the population [71]. This mechanism can induce the production of virulence factors and mechanisms of resistance to antibiotics [72]. Interestingly, AIP with a structure different from that produced by the same strain may excerpt an inhibitory effect on the Agr system, instead of the cognate autoinducing function [70]. *S. aureus* requires the Agr system to be able to adapt to changes in the environment during growth to regulate the bacteria's virulence factors [70]. The Agr system has two adjacent transcriptional regions, named RNAII and RNAIII, its expression is regulated by P2 and P3 promoters. Regarding the RNAII region, it is known that it is an operon of four genes (*agrBDCA*), which is responsible for encoding the mechanism of the *quorum sensing* system [73]. The RNAIII transcript is the main effector molecule, and its function is to regulate the expression of most of the target genes that depend on the Agr system (**Figure 1**) [69].

AgrB is a membrane endopeptidase whose function is to cleave the mature AIP from the AIP precursor (AgrD), to form the macrocyclic thiolactone structure and release it into the cytoplasm [70]. AIP interacts with AgrC, a membrane-bound histidine receptor kinase, which subsequently phosphorylates AgrA in the cytoplasm [74]; once phosphorylated, AgrA joins P2 and P3, regulating RNAII and III transcription [73].

AgrA also acts by inducing the expression of phenol-soluble modulins (PSMs). The RNAIII gene encodes a small RNA molecule that is the main effector molecule of the quorum sensing system that is responsible for increasing the expression of cell surface proteins. Four groups of Agr are known in *S. aureus* called agr I-IV each producing a distinctive AIP structure [73]. The Agr system produces increased expression of enzymes and toxins such as serine proteases, DNase, toxic shock toxin-1 (TSST-1),

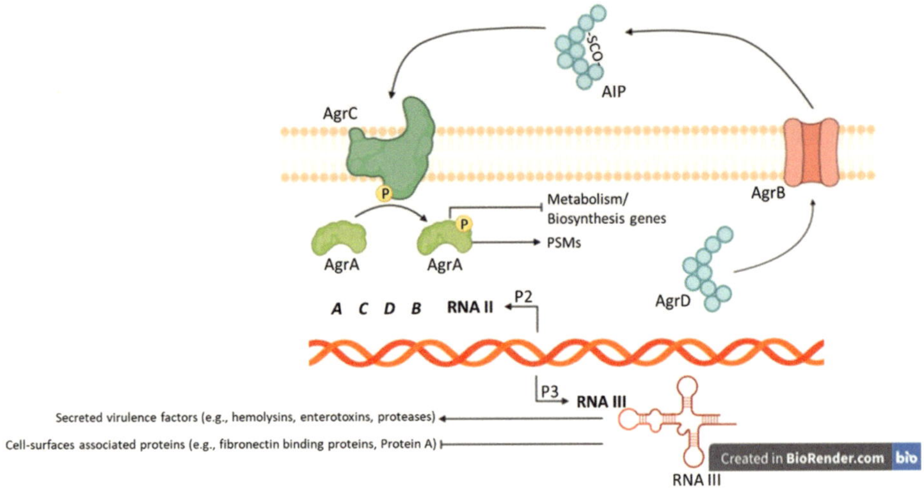

Figure 1.
The Agr system can regulate the virulence of S. aureus. The activation of the system is carried out by an autoinducing peptide (AIP), which accumulates extracellularly when reaching a critical concentration or depletion of glucose. Agr system has two adjacent transcriptional regions (RNAII and RNAIII), and its expression is mediated by the promoters P2 and P3. The RNAII transcript is encoded by the agrBDCA operon, which is the main part of the system, while the RNAIII transcript is the main effector molecule and is responsible for regulating the expression of most Agr-dependent target genes. RNAIII contains the hld (hemolysin δ) genes and leads to the expression and secretion of virulence factors (hemolysins, proteases, enterotoxins, etc.), it is also responsible for inhibiting the expression of cell surface proteins. (modified from Salam and Quave [73].

fibrinolysin, and enterotoxin B and also regulates the expression of colonization and biofilm formation factors [75].

During infectious processes, *S. aureus* produces a large number of enzymes, including lipases, proteases, and elastases, which serve to invade and damage host tissues. This bacterium can produce septic shock, and some strains produce superantigens, causing various intoxications, such as toxic shock syndrome and food poisoning. Some strains produce exfoliative toxins and epidermolysins that can cause bullous impetigo or scalded skin syndrome [76].

During the pathogenesis of *S. aureus*, it is essential to carry out the regulation of the expression of virulence factors. This regulation occurs in a coordinated manner during the bacterial infection. MSCRAMM expression generally occurs during the logarithmic phase of growth, whereas toxins are synthesized during the stationary phase. For the infectious process, the early expression of the MSCRAMM proteins is required, which promotes the initial colonization of the tissues, while later the synthesis of toxins that are secreted by the bacteria and that can cause direct damage to the host, this facilitates the spread and persistence of bacteria in the host [76, 77].

Although Agr system is one of the most important studied virulence factor regulation mechanisms, there are several other global regulators of virulence gene transcription that function in a complex network to regulate virulence. Some of these regulatory systems are *sar*, *sae*, *srr*, *sigB*, *rot*, and *mgr loci*, among others, and form a complex regulatory network controlling virulence [78]. With the advent of whole genome sequencing techniques in addition to the accumulating knowledge of virulence gene regulation and functions, attempts have been proposed to construct system biology tools to predict virulence of *S. aureus* strains from genomic sequence [79]. Although there is the great amount of information on *S. aureus* pathotypes and genomic sequence, this goal is still far to be reached due to the complexity of the virulence regulatory network in *S. aureus*.

2.2 Biofilms

2.2.1 Polysaccharide intercellular adhesion (PIA)

Polysaccharide of intercellular adhesion (PIA) or poly-N-acetylglucosamine (PNAG) is a fundamental biofilm exopolysaccharide and constitutes most of the extracellular matrix of staphylococcal biofilms [71].

The PIA is constituted by the linear polysaccharide of poly-β(1-6)-N-acetylglucosamine and allows the mediation of bacterial intercellular adhesion; in addition, it forms the structure of the biofilm and bacterial adhesion on surfaces, in addition to protection against host defenses [75]. This is because PIA generates positive charges around the surface of bacteria (which are negatively charged by WTA), triggering electrostatic interactions that allow them to adhere to cells and tissues [71]. PIA is synthesized by the *icaADBC* locus, which is part of the accessory genes on plasmids, and therefore not all *S. aureus* strains have it [75]. However, PIA is so far the only important element involved in biofilm generation in vivo [80], but it does not appear in all isolates from biofilm-associated *S. aureus* infections, so other proteins are involved in its formation (SasG, SpA, Fnbp, among others) [26].

Figure 2 shows that the structure of the *icaADBC* locus, *icaA* (N-acetylglucosaminyltransferase) encodes a very important transmembrane protein in the synthesis of the poly-N-acetylglucosamine polymer, being more efficient with polymer residues of more than twenty, and is only synthesized together with the *icaD* gene protein. Both proteins (*icaA* and *icaD*) are essential in the synthesis of exopolysaccharides. The third gene, *icaC*, translocates the poly-N-acetylglucosamine polymer to the cell surface, and the product of the *icaB* gene produces its deacetylation; this is very important for the structural maturation of the exopolysaccharide biofilm and allows the adhesion of the polymer with the surface of the bacteria [75, 82]. *icaR* is the fifth gene of the *icaADBC* locus, and it is transcribed in the opposite direction to the aforementioned genes, the start codon between *icaR* and *icaA* is separated by 163 bp (**Figure 2**). The role of *icaR* is to be a negative regulator of the *icaADBC* locus of *S. aureus*, and it encodes a 22 kDa protein of the TetR family. Otherwise, *icaZ* has only been found in strains of *S. epidermidis*, and its expression depends on the conditions of the medium and the incubation temperature [82, 83].

The *icaR* gene is responsible for the expression of the *ica* locus and in turn is regulated by the SarA and σB stress sigma systems (**Figure 3**). SarA belongs to the family of staphylococcal regular accessory proteins (Sar) and functions as an activator or repressor of the transcription of various *S. aureus* genes involved in its pathogenicity, so SarA is a virulence factor of great importance. The *agr* locus is regulated by SarA [78]. The Agr system regulates the change in expression of cell surface proteins in the early phases of bacterial growth (latency and exponential phase), to the synthesis of degrading proteins and toxins (post-exponential and stationary phase). The ability of *S. aureus* to form biofilms can be reduced by expression of the *agr* locus [75, 80, 82].

The formation of biofilms is generated from a complex production of extracellular polymeric molecules, such as amyloid fibrils, extracellular DNA, and phenol-soluble modulins (PSM), and this is due to the synthesis of nucleases, proteases, and PSM peptides [84]. The presence of PSM is highly regulated by Agr, this could indicate that

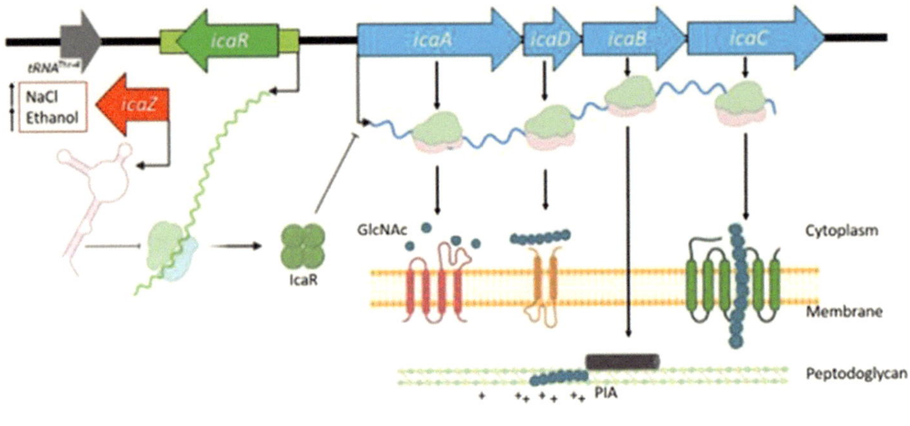

Figure 2.
Structure of the icaADBC locus. Organization of the locus in S. epidermidis RP62A. Colored arrows indicate the coding regions. icaA encodes the enzyme N-acetylglucosaminyl-transferase (membrane protein), icaC is responsible for the translocation of the poly-N-acetylglucosamine polymer to the surface of the bacteria, in the case of icaB, it deacetylates the polymer. icaR is transcribed in the opposite direction with respect to the mentioned genes, and its function is to regulate the operon and therefore the biofilm. icaZ has only been reported in S. epidermidis under some environmental and temperature conditions (modified from Lerch et al. [81]).

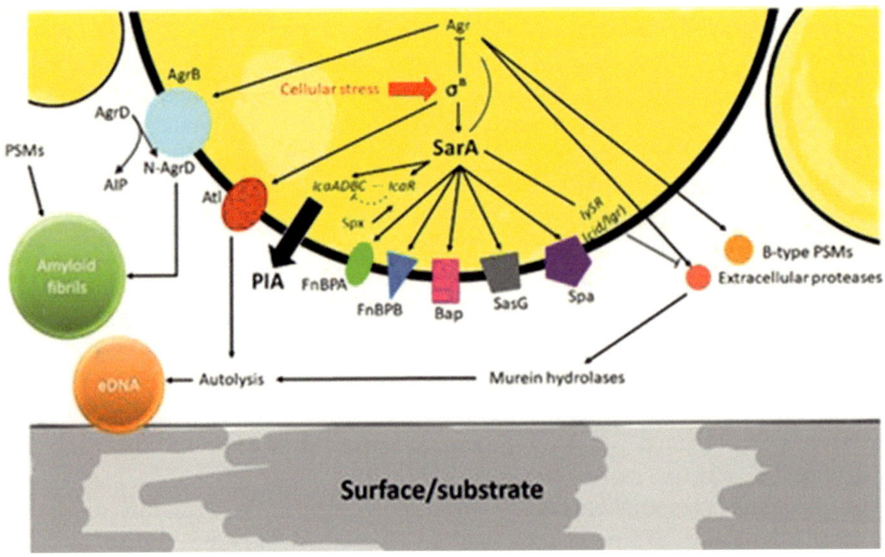

Figure 3.
Diagram of the interactions that favor the formation and degradation of biofilms. The anabolic phase of biofilm formation is shown on the left side of the figure, where several critical extracellular polymeric substances (EPS): PIA, amyloid fibrils, and eDNA, are present. Also shown is the lytSR operon with its lrg/cid target genes. Membrane protein components involved in biofilm formation are shown in the center of the figure, including FnBP adhesins, biofilm-associated protein (Bap), Spa, and SasG. On the right side, the molecules of the catabolic processes of the biofilm are shown, including extracellular proteins and PSM. The Agr system, the σB factor, and SarA are the main regulators, modifying bacterial behavior in response to various environmental stimuli (modified from Arciola et al. [75]).

the biofilm formation processes that depend on the Agr system are due to the expression of PSM [77]. The mechanisms of sessile and planktonic phenotypes require sensitive coordinated and efficient control during the invasive phase of bacteria [75].

There is evidence that *S. epidermidis icaA* (+) overexpresses the biofilm formation phenotype under *in vitro* conditions. However, *S. aureus* makes it different since the positive strains of the *ica* locus are not always expressed *in vitro* and do not need anaerobiosis or medium supplementation with other nutrients to express it. In contrast, *S. aureus* strains have higher biofilm production under *in vivo* conditions. Some stress-induced conditions *in vitro*, such as starvation, iron limitation, non-inhibitory concentrations of ethanol, heat stress, NaCl, and various antibiotics, have been reported to increase biofilm production [75].

2.2.2 Amyloid proteins

The stability of the biofilm is due to the presence of amyloid proteins [85]. The amyloid structure is composed of three packed β-fibers that are resistant to denaturing conditions and are not degraded by proteases [86].

Amyloid proteins can bind to eDNA and function as inters fibrils in the biofilm, functioning as a solid bond, which allows the bacteria to wait for the environmental conditions to improve to favor their dissociation and allow the dispersion of the biofilm [85]. PSMs are necessary to increase the volume, roughness, thickness, and channel formation in the biofilm [87]. These surfactant peptides (PSM) play a fundamental function in the three-dimensional structure of the biofilm, in addition to favoring its detachment [87], and are determinants of biofilm maturation in vivo [71, 82]. **Figure 4** shows a diagram of the main components expressed by *S. aureus* in the formation of biofilms.

2.2.3 Fibrin biofilm

S. aureus can survive in the blood due to the production of the enzyme coagulase (CoA), which is regulated by the SaeRS two-component system. Detection of enzyme activity (Coa or staphylocoagulase) is very common in the clinical laboratory to identify strains of *S. aureus* from other staphylococci [89]. Highly relevant in the development of biofilms is *coa* gene, under natural conditions and is present in 100% of *S. aureus* strains. After maturation, fibrin-coated biofilms have increased defense and resistance against antibiotics [88].

Coa function is activated by binding to prothrombin from the blood, allowing the formation of the active staphylothrombin complex that converts soluble fibrinogen to insoluble fibrin, which is used by *S. aureus* to reinforce the biofilm. Whether S. *aureus* can form biofilms mediated by the *coa* gene depends on contact of bacterial cells with the host cell surface, and an important protein for this binding is ClfA [90].

There are indications that the colonization of medical devices by *S. aureus* is due to the production of fibrin biofilms mediated by the *coa* gene; however, over longer periods of time, other adhesins that also form biofilms play a more important role in their maturation [88]. Zapotoczna et al. [91] observe that after 24 h of fibrin biofilm formation, they became weaker in the presence of antibiotics compared with biofilms of another protein composition (e.g., FnBP) in the same period of development; however, with the passage of time, the fibrin biofilms became more resistant.

2.3 Biofilm formation

Upon initial contact, a planktonic cell can reversibly associate with a surface, and if the cell does not detach, then it will irreversibly bind to it [25, 27].

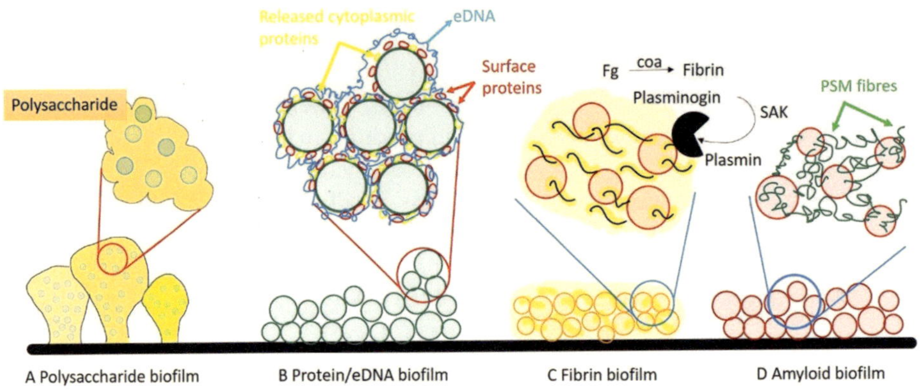

Figure 4.
Main types of biofilms. A: PIA/PNAG polysaccharide biofilm by strains with the icaADBC operon (common in MRSA), B: surface proteins (BAP, FnBP, and SasG), interact between cells during biofilm formation. eDNA and cytoplasmic proteins diffused after lysis participate as elements of the biofilm matrix, C: coagulase-mediated activation of fibrinogen (Fg) into fibrin, which is activated to strengthen the biofilm, which can be dissociated by the plasmin produced post-staphylokinase (SAK) (plasminogen-mediated), D: PSMs have surface-active properties that promote biofilm breakdown and, in turn, can accumulate as amyloid aggregates (modified from Zapotoczna et al. [88]).

When *S. aureus* adheres to host cells and tissues or to the surface of prosthetic materials, it can reproduce, colonize, and persist in these sites, in a variety of ways [76]. The first of the mechanisms used by bacteria is the formation of biofilms, *S. aureus* can form them on the surface of tissues, thereby colonizing and persisting in tissues, in addition to evading some of the host's immune mechanisms, also to blocking the role of antibiotics [92].

The biofilm is defined as a set of aggregated bacteria and is made up of cells adhered to each other (sessile cells). The cells are located within a matrix with extracellular polymeric substances (proteins, exopolysaccharides, adhesins, eDNA, etc.), which present an altered phenotype of growth, genetic expression, and protein production [92, 93], with respect to normal cells, normal planktonic (free life) [90]. Biofilms can form on biotic and abiotic surfaces, and those bacteria that are coated within the biofilm are 10–1000 times less sensitive to antibiotics than planktonic bacterial cells [71, 94, 95].

The formation of biofilms has been described through a cycle from the study of different bacterial species and is composed of (1) reversible adhesion, (2) irreversible union (formation of microcolonies), (3) maturation, and (4) dispersion [71, 96]. **Figure 5** shows a schematic of the biofilm formation cycle. However, in 2014, Moormeier et al. [23] proposed five stages in the formation of biofilms for *S. aureus*: (1) fixation, (2) multiplication, (3) exodus, (4) maturation, and (5) dispersion. The first stage of biofilm formation was mentioned in the section on adhesins.

2.3.1 Components of the biofilm matrix

2.3.1.1 Extracellular DNA (eDNA)

When the biofilm is formed, the extracellular matrix (ECM) is produced, made up of polysaccharides, proteins, and/or extracellular DNA, which confers the three-dimensional structure that stabilizes and matures the biofilm [97]. The hypothetical

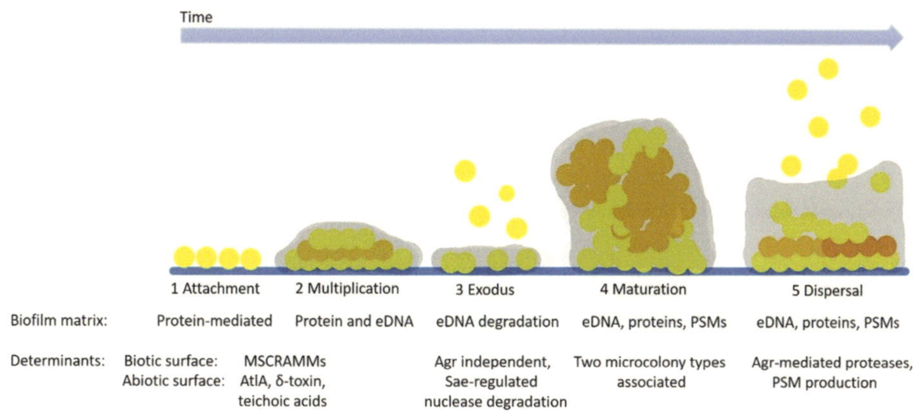

Figure 5.
The five parts of S. aureus biofilm formation. The process of biofilm formation can be explained in five main stages: (1) initial attachment or binding, (2) multiplication, (3) exodus or primary migration, (4) maturation, and (5) dispersal. 1. S. aureus Binds to a surface (abiotic or biotic) via MSCRAMM or nonpolar interactions. 2. Once cells adhere, a biofilm is formed, which is a confluent layer of cells, eDNA, and protein matrix. 3. When confluence is reached, cell exodus occurs, releasing a small number of cells from the biofilm by degradation of nuclease enzymes to eDNA (regulated by Sae), which allows the development of microcolonies in the biofilm space. 4. These microcolonies are formed from cellular sources that remain attached in the exodus stage. This stage consists of accelerated cell division that forms protein aggregates, including eDNA and PSM. 5. Quorum sensing by the Agr system initiates regulation of the biofilm matrix and cell dispersal through activation of proteases and/or PSM (modified from Moormier et al. [26]).

mechanism of eDNA adhesion postulates that eDNA is adsorbed on the membrane of individual bacteria in long loop structures measuring up to 300 nm [98]. It has also been described that DNA loops interact with rough surfaces at the nanoscale, which increases the bacterial adhesion surface to this type of surface (**Figure 5**) [99].

eDNA favors the hydrophobicity of the bacterial surface, single-stranded DNA has amphiphilic properties, the hydrophilic part for deoxyribose, and the hydrophobic part for nitrogenous bases. Otherwise, double-stranded DNA hybridizes with each other by hydrogen bonds (Watson-Crick bonds) and hydrophobic interactions. Various studies have reported that eDNA increases the hydrophobicity of bacteria. Das et al. [100] reported that the presence of eDNA increases the adhesion of bacterial cells on hydrophobic surfaces (**Figure 6**) [99].

eDNA also favors resistance to antimicrobial drugs by inducing the expression of resistance genes. eDNA can form complexes with divalent metal cations (Mg^{2+}, Ca^{2+}, Mn^{2+}, and Zn^{2+}), which neutralizes the negative charge on the outer part of the bacterial membrane and increases its resistance to host antimicrobial peptides and cationic antibiotics such as aminoglycosides. However, eDNA can induce immune system activation, although the biofilm protects bacteria from some processes such as phagocytosis [99].

How components of the biofilm matrix are externalized is still not fully understood. Mutant strains defective in autolysis have been reported to have poor biofilm-forming capacity compared with strains that do not produce PIA biofilms [94]. Phagocytosis-mediated cell death is another mechanism of eDNA release and lysis-independent methods such as specialized secretion or vesicle formation [101, 102].

2.3.2 Biofilm multiplication stage

After bacterial attachment to a surface and under sufficient nutritional conditions, adherent *S. aureus* cells can multiply and accumulate. However, newly divided cells

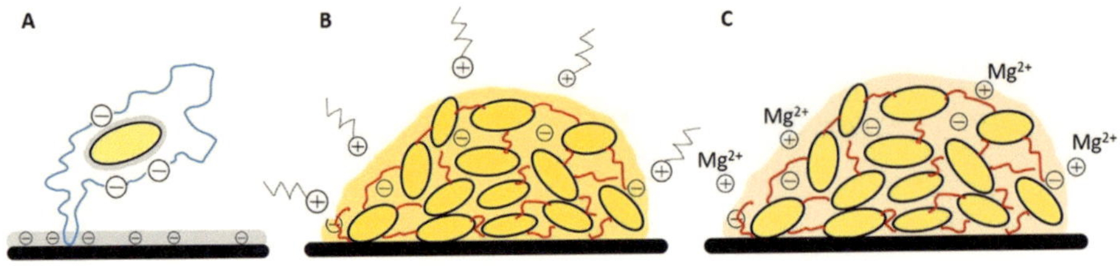

Figure 6.
Functions of extracellular DNA. (A) eDNA aids adhesion on surfaces by penetrating the electrically repulsive double layer. Acid-base interactions lead to bacterial adhesion. (B) eDNA generates chelating complexes with cationic antimicrobial peptides of the host's innate immune system. (C) eDNA generates complexes with divalent cations, triggering a response in the bacteria that increases pathogenicity and antimicrobial resistance (modified from Okshevsky et al. [99]).

are very susceptible to detachment, primarily from fluid flow. To maintain immature biofilm stability, *S. aureus* can produce a wide range of molecules that stabilize intracellular interactions. This process is called the multiplication stage [26].

Staphylococci strains can produce a wide range of extracellular proteins (CWA, FnBP, SdrC, and ClfB), which promote biofilm formation by favoring intercellular binding, once they are attached to the surface through a dual role in the stage's union and accumulation. But there is evidence that they are also involved during the multiplication stage of biofilm development [23]. PIA functions as a component of ECM in the early stages of *S. aureus* biofilm formation [26].

Foulston et al. [103] showed that the enzymes enolase and glyceraldehyde 3-phosphate dehydrogenase (GAPDH) (which is not a biofilm-forming protein) can be activated as a component of the ECM in response to a decrease in pH, around the biofilm (**Figure** 7). This would imply that under acidic conditions, enolase and GAPDH can bind to eDNA [104]. Otherwise, it has been reported that other extracellular proteins such as PSM, β-hemolysin (Hlb), and IsaB (immunodominant surface antigen B) bind to eDNA to stabilize the ECM [26].

2.3.3 Biofilm exodus stage

In time-lapse microscopic observations of biofilms, a phase was found that was termed "Exodus," due to a clear coordinated cell release around 6 h after the start of the multiplication stage, which is an early dispersal event that occurs at the same time as the formation of the microcolony and produces the restructuring of the biofilm (**Figure** 7). The exodus phase is determined by the degradation of eDNA by nucleases and does not depend on the Agr system, which is produced after the development of the microcolony. The degradation of eDNA in the ECM by endogenous nucleases decreases the total biomass of the biofilm [23, 24, 83, 105]. The exodus phase is highly regulated, since only a part of the bacterial cells in the biofilm presents the expression of the *nuc* gene (which encodes a thermonuclease, used as an identification criterion for *S. aureus*), which favors the shedding of most of the cell population of the biofilm formed [36]. Also, Moormeier et al. [23] noted changes important in ECM as the biofilm structure advances, initially only consisting of membrane protein components (binding and multiplication phase), to relying on eDNA and proteins released to the outside (exodus stage). Therefore, a biofilm is only composed of PIA, protein, and eDNA must be replaced by a more complex model of biofilm development and ECM composition over time as the biofilm forms [26]. Therefore, the reduction of the

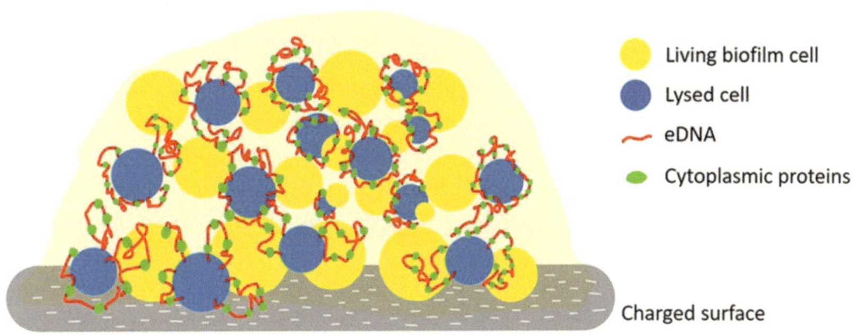

Figure 7.
Scheme of intercellular interactions in the biofilm multiplication stage. Early in biofilm development, free-living (planktonic) cells adhere to surfaces through electrostatic interactions mediated by teichoic acids, PSM, autolysin A, etc. As the multiplication stage progresses, some cells die or lyse (blue circles) releasing cytoplasmic proteins (green circles) and eDNA (red lines) into the extracellular medium, enveloping living bacteria (yellow circles) in a mixture of DNA and proteins cytoplasmic (modified from Moormeier et al. [23]).

bacterial population at the beginning of biofilm formation (by death or exodus) is an important requirement for its maturation. It has been observed that when there is no exodus phase, as is the case with *S. aureus* strains that have mutations in the *nuc* gene, the formation of microcolonies does not occur [23].

2.3.4 Biofilm maturation stage

The formation of microcolony structures is essential in the biofilm maturation process, since they provide a larger contact surface for obtaining nutrients and eliminating waste, in addition to favoring the dispersion of bacterial cells within the biofilm. Research carried out on other species of bacteria has reported the development of microcolony-like structures during the biofilm formation stages of *S. aureus* [23, 87, 106], the mechanism of its formation is not known.

A previously described model [87] mentions that the formation of microcolonies in the development of the biofilm is a subtractive process, in which channels are formed in it due to the dispersion caused by the PSM. However, in microscopy observations at different times, it has been described that microcolonies are formed from different cell foci of the basal layer once the exodus phase begins (**Figure 5**).

After the maturation stage, the release of bacteria from the interior of the biofilm occurs through dispersion, which reactivates the free-living state of the bacterial cell (planktonic state) [93, 107]. DNase I has been reported to be an inhibitor of PIA-independent biofilm development in MRSA strains of clinical isolates; however, it does not inhibit PIA-dependent MSSA strains [104]. In the same investigation, DNase I effectively inhibited biofilm development of MRSA strains, but failed to destroy already formed biofilms [108, 109].

2.3.5 Biofilm dispersion stage

Dispersion processes are fundamental in the composition of the biofilm, since through these the cells are released from the biofilm individually or in large groups of bacteria, if there are favorable environmental conditions. This is very important in biofilm-associated infections, as they facilitate systemic spread, and it has been shown that cells shed from biofilms from medical devices and catheters can cause endocarditis or sepsis [71, 80].

Mechanisms influencing the control of biofilm scattering have been studied and reported to be mediated by Agr quorum sensing control [84]. In the dispersion stage, the bacteria of the outermost layers of the biofilm are responsible for the expression of the *agr* genes, which leads to the detachment of the cells, and at the same time the renewal of the biofilm; however, *agr* genes are also expressed by bacteria in the inner part of the biofilm, where it is used for channel formation [70, 87, 110].

Some toxins influence the development of biofilms. For example, α-hemolysin (Hla) and leukocidin AB (LukAB) are involved in biofilm persistence [111]; Hla and LukAB are also synergistically involved in promoting macrophage dysfunction and death. Dastgheyb et al. [112] showed that PSMs block biofilm formation by disrupting interactions between ECM molecules with the bacterial surface. Perasamy et al. [87] reported similar results regarding the influence of the PSMs of *S. aureus* with the development of the biofilm, and that PSM degraded it, which produced its early dispersion due to the surfactant properties of the toxin [113].

The importance of the Agr system is essential for cell communication within the biofilm formed, to form and establish the three-dimensional structure by controlling cell dispersion. However, Agr system does not regulate other adhesive molecules of biofilm formation, as is the case with PIA [75].

3. Conclusions

S. aureus is a highly relevant pathogenic bacterium for humans and other mammals, since it can bind very intensely to different components of the extracellular matrix and thus infect cells. It also has mechanisms that allow it to colonize, persist, and survive in unfavorable environmental conditions for growth, such is the case of the formation of biofilms, which allows it to evade various human immune mechanisms very efficiently. The complex and dynamic composition of *S. aureus* biofilms, as well as the existence of a complex genetic regulatory network driving biofilm formation and maturation, offer a wide variety of potential pharmacological targets for the control of *S. aureus* infections.

Conflict of interest

The authors declare no conflict of interest.

Author details

Samuel González-García[1], Aída Hamdan-Partida[2], Juan José Valdez-Alarcón[3], Anaid Bustos-Hamdan[4] and Jaime Bustos-Martínez[2*]

1 Doctorate in Biological and Health Sciences, Autonomous Metropolitan University, Mexico City, Mexico

2 Department of Health Care, Autonomous Metropolitan University-Xochimilco, Mexico City, Mexico

3 Faculty of Veterinary Medicine and Zootechnics, Multidisciplinary Center for Studies in Biotechnology, Universidad Michoacana de San Nicolás de Hidalgo, Michoacán, Mexico

4 National Institute of Perinatology "Isidro Espinosa de los Reyes", Mexico City, Mexico

*Address all correspondence to: jbustos@correo.xoc.uam.mx

References

[1] Barrera-Rivas CI, Valle-Hurtado NA, González-Luego GM, Baizabal-Aguirre VM, Bravo-Patiño A, Cajero-Juárez M, et al. Bacteriophage therapy: An alternative for the treatment of *Staphylococcus aureus* infections in animals and animal models. In: Frontiers in *Staphylococcus aureus*. London, UK: IntechOpen; 2017. pp. 179-201. DOI: 10.5772/65761

[2] Danelli T, Duarte FC, de Oliveira TA, da Silva RS, Frizon-Alfieri D, Goncalves GB, et al. Nasal carriage by *Staphylococcus aureus* among healthcare workers and students attending a University Hospital in Southern Brazil: Prevalence, phenotypic, and molecular characteristics. Interdisciplinary Perspectives on Infectious Diseases. 2020;**2020**:3808036. DOI: 10.1155/2020/3808036

[3] Wertheim HF, Melles DC, Vos MC, van Leeuwen W, van Belkum A, Verbrugh HA, et al. The role of nasal carriage in *Staphylococcus aureus* infections. The Lancet Infectious Diseases. 2005;**5**:751-762. DOI: 10.1016/S1473-3099(05)70295-4

[4] Roghmann MC, Johnson JK, Stine OC, Lydecker AD, Ryan KA, Mitchell BD, et al. Persistent *Staphylococcus aureus* colonization is not a strongly heritable trait in Amish families. PLoS One. 2011;**6**:e17368. DOI: 10.1371/journal.pone.0017368

[5] Sollid JUE, Furberg AS, Hanssen AM, Johannessen M. *Staphylococcus aureus*: Determinants of human carriage. Infection, Genetics and Evolution. 2014;**21**:531-541. DOI: 10.1016/j.meegid.2013.03.020

[6] Mertz D, Frei R, Jaussi B, Tietz A, Stebler C, Flückiger U, et al. Throat swabs are necessary to reliably detect carriers of *Staphylococcus aureus*. Clinical Infectious Diseases. 2007;**4**:475-477. DOI: 10.1086/520016

[7] González-García S, Hamdan-Partida A, Bustos-Hamdan A, Bustos-Martínez J. Factors of nasopharynx that favor the colonization and persistence of *Staphylococcus aureus*. In: Zhou X, Zhang Z, editors. Pharynx—Diagnosis and Treatment. London: IntechOpen; 2021. pp. 1-21. DOI: 10.5772/intechopen.95843

[8] Leonard AC, Petrie LE, Cox G. Bacterial anti-adhesives: Inhibition of *Staphylococcus aureus* nasal colonization. ACS Infectious Diseases. 2019;**5**:1668-1681. DOI: 10.1021/acsinfecdis.9b00193

[9] Brown AF, Leech JM, Rogers TR, McLoughlin RM. *Staphylococcus aureus* colonization: Modulation of host immune response and impact on human vaccine design. Frontiers in Immunology. 2014;**4**:507. DOI: 10.3389/fimmu.2013.00507

[10] Kim SJ, Chang J, Rimal B, Yang H, Schaefer J. Surface proteins and the formation of biofilms by *Staphylococcus aureus*. Biochimica et Biophysica Acta—Biomembranes. 2018;**3**:749-756. DOI: 10.1016/j.bbamem.2017.12.003

[11] Mistretta N, Brossaud M, Telles F, Sanchez V, Talaga P, Rokbi B. Glycosylation of *Staphylococcus aureus* cell wall teichoic acid is influenced by environmental conditions. Scientific Reports. 2019;**9**:1-11. DOI: 10.1038/s41598-019-39929-1

[12] Winstel V, Kühner P, Salomon F, Larsen J, Skov R, Hoffmann W, et al. Wall teichoic acid glycosylation governs

Staphylococcus aureus nasal colonization. mBio. 2015;**4**:e00632-e00615. DOI: 10.1128/mBio.00632-15

[13] Brown S, Santa Maria Jr JP, Walker S. Wall teichoic acids of gram-positive bacteria. Annual Review of Microbiology. 2013;**67**:313-336. DOI: 10.1146/annurev-micro-092412-155620

[14] Baur S, Rautenberg M, Faulstich M, Grau T, Severin Y, Unger C, et al. A nasal epithelial receptor for *Staphylococcus aureus* WTA governs adhesion to epithelial cells and modulates nasal colonization. PLoS Pathogens. 2014;**5**:e1004089. DOI: 10.1371/journal.ppat.1004089

[15] Misawa Y, Kelley KA, Wang X, Wang L, Park WB, Birtel J, et al. *Staphylococcus aureus* colonization of the mouse gastrointestinal tract is modulated by wall teichoic acid, capsule, and surface proteins. PLoS Pathogens. 2015;**7**:e1005061. DOI: 10.1371/journal.ppat.1005061

[16] Wanner S, Schade J, Keinhörster D, Weller N, George SE, Kull L, et al. Wall teichoic acids mediate increased virulence in *Staphylococcus aureus*. Nature Microbiology. 2017;**4**:1-12. DOI: 10.1038/nmicrobiol.2016.257

[17] Winstel V, Sanchez-Carballo P, Holst O, Xia G, Peschel A. Biosynthesis of the unique wall teichoic acid of *Staphylococcus aureus* lineage ST395. mBio. 2014;**2**:e00869-e00814. DOI: 10.1128/mBio.00869-14

[18] Suzuki T, Swoboda JG, Campbell J, Walker S, Gilmore MS. In vitro antimicrobial activity of wall teichoic acid biosynthesis inhibitors against *Staphylococcus aureus* isolates. Antimicrobial Agents and Chemotherapy. 2011;**2**:767-774. DOI: 10.1128/AAC.00879-10

[19] Weidenmaier C, Kokai-Kun JF, Kulauzovic E, Kohler T, Thumm G, Stoll H, et al. Differential roles of sortase-anchored surface proteins and wall teichoic acid in *Staphylococcus aureus* nasal colonization. International Journal of Medical Microbiology. 2008;**5-6**:505-513. DOI: 10.1016/j.ijmm.2007.11.006

[20] Weidenmaier C, Goerke C, Wolz C. *Staphylococcus aureus* determinants for nasal colonization. Trends in Microbiology. 2012;**5**:243-250. DOI: 10.1016/j.tim.2012.03.004

[21] Burian M, Wolz C, Goerke C. Regulatory adaptation of *Staphylococcus aureus* during nasal colonization of humans. PLoS One. 2010;**4**:e10040. DOI: 10.1371/journal.pone.0010040

[22] Burian M, Rautenberg M, Kohler T, Fritz M, Krismer B, Unger C, et al. Temporal expression of adhesion factors and activity of global regulators during establishment of *Staphylococcus aureus* nasal colonization. The Journal of Infectious Diseases. 2010;**9**:1414-1421. DOI: 10.1086/651619

[23] Moormeier DE, Bose JL, Horswill AR, Bayles KW. Temporal and stochastic control of *Staphylococcus aureus* biofilm development. mBio. 2014;**5**:e01341-e01314. DOI: 10.1128/mBio.01341-14

[24] Kurokawa K, Takahashi K, Lee BL. The staphylococcal surface-glycopolymer wall teichoic acid (WTA) is crucial for complement activation and immunological defense against *Staphylococcus aureus* infection. Immunobiology. 2016;**10**:1091-1101. DOI: 10.1016/j.imbio.2016.06.003

[25] Foster TJ, Geoghegan JA, Ganesh VK, Höök M. Adhesion, invasion and evasion: The many functions of the surface proteins of *Staphylococcus aureus*. Nature

Reviews. Microbiology. 2014;**1**:49-62. DOI: 10.1038/nrmicro3161

[26] Moormeier DE, Bayles KW. *Staphylococcus aureus* biofilm: A complex developmental organism. Molecular Microbiology. 2017;**3**:365-376. DOI: 10.1111/mmi.13634

[27] Kong C, Chee CF, Richter K, Thomas N, Rahman NA, Nathan S. Suppression of *Staphylococcus aureus* biofilm formation and virulence by a benzimidazole derivative, UM-C162. Scientific Reports. 2018;**1**:1-16. DOI: 10.1038/s41598-018-21141-2

[28] Ganesh VK, Barbu EM, Deivanayagam CC, Le B, Anderson AS, Matsuka YV, et al. Structural and biochemical characterization of *Staphylococcus aureus* clumping factor B/ligand interactions. The Journal of Biological Chemistry. 2011;**29**:25963-25972. DOI: 10.1074/jbc.M110.217414

[29] Lacey KA, Mulcahy ME, Towell AM, Geoghegan JA, McLoughlin RM. Clumping factor B is an important virulence factor during *Staphylococcus aureus* skin infection and a promising vaccine target. PLoS Pathogens. 2019;**4**:e1007713. DOI: 10.1371/journal.ppat.1007713

[30] Abraham NM, Jefferson KK. *Staphylococcus aureus* clumping factor B mediates biofilm formation in the absence of calcium. Microbiology. 2012;**158**(Pt 6):1504. DOI: 10.1099/mic.0.057018-0

[31] Mulcahy ME, Geoghegan JA, Monk IR, O'Keeffe KM, Walsh EJ, Foster TJ, et al. Nasal colonisation by *Staphylococcus aureus* depends upon clumping factor B binding to the squamous epithelial cell envelope protein loricrin. PLoS Pathogens. 2012;**12**:e1003092. DOI: 10.1371/journal.ppat.1003092

[32] Hait JM, Cao G, Kastanis G, Yin L, Pettengill JB, Tallent SM. Evaluation of virulence determinants using whole-genome sequencing and phenotypic biofilm analysis of outbreak-linked *Staphylococcus aureus* isolates. Frontiers in Microbiology. 2021;**12**:687625. DOI: 10.3389/fmicb.2021.687625

[33] Hamdan-Partida A, González-García S, de la Rosa GE, Bustos-Martínez J. Community-acquired methicillin-resistant *Staphylococcus aureus* can persist in the throat. International Journal of Medical Microbiology. 2018;**4**:469-475. DOI: 10.1016/j.ijmm.2018.04.002

[34] Lacey KA, Geoghegan JA, McLoughlin RM. The role of *Staphylococcus aureus* virulence factors in skin infection and their potential as vaccine antigens. Pathogens. 2016;**1**:22. DOI: 10.3390/pathogens5010022

[35] Fleury OM, McAleer MA, Feuillie C, Formosa-Dague C, Sansevere E, Bennett DE, et al. Clumping factor B promotes adherence of *Staphylococcus aureus* to corneocytes in atopic dermatitis. Infection and Immunity. 2017;**6**:e00994-e00916. DOI: 10.1128/IAI.00994-16

[36] McAleese FM, Walsh EJ, Sieprawska M, Potempa J, Foster TJ. Loss of clumping factor B fibrinogen binding activity by *Staphylococcus aureus* involves cessation of transcription, shedding and cleavage by metalloprotease. The Journal of Biological Chemistry. 2001;**32**:29969-29978. DOI: 10.1074/jbc.M102389200

[37] Ngo QV, Faass L, Sähr A, Hildebrand D, Eigenbrod T, Heeg K, et al. Inflammatory response against *Staphylococcus aureus* via intracellular sensing of nucleic acids in keratinocytes. Frontiers in Immunology. 2022;**13**:1-12. DOI: 10.3389/fimmu.2022.828626

[38] Pi Y, Chen W, Ji Q. Structural basis of *Staphylococcus aureus* surface protein SdrC. Biochemistry. 2020;**15**:1465-1469. DOI: 10.1021/acs.biochem.0c00124

[39] Vitry P, Valotteau C, Feuillie C, Bernard S, Alsteens D, Geoghegan JA, et al. Force-induced strengthening of the interaction between *Staphylococcus aureus* clumping factor B and loricrin. mBio. 2017;**6**:e01748-e01717. DOI: 10.1128/mBio.01748-17

[40] Liu H, Lv J, Qi X, Ding Y, Li D, Hu L, et al. The carriage of the serine-aspartate repeat protein-encoding *sdr* genes among *Staphylococcus aureus* lineages. The Brazilian Journal of Infectious Diseases. 2015;**5**:498-502. DOI: 10.1016/j.bjid.2015.07.003

[41] Askarian F, Ajayi C, Hanssen AM, Van Sorge NM, Pettersen I, Diep DB, et al. The interaction between *Staphylococcus aureus* SdrD and desmoglein 1 is important for adhesion to host cells. Scientific Reports. 2016;**1**:1-11. DOI: 10.1038/srep22134

[42] Sharp JA, Echague CG, Hair PS, Ward MD, Nyalwidhe JO, Geoghegan JA, et al. *Staphylococcus aureus* surface protein SdrE binds complement regulator factor H as an immune evasion tactic. PLoS One. 2012;**5**:e38407. DOI: 10.1371/journal.pone.0038407

[43] Hair PS, Foley CK, Krishna NK, Nyalwidhe JO, Geoghegan JA, Foster TJ, et al. Complement regulator C4BP binds to *Staphylococcus aureus* surface proteins SdrE and Bbp inhibiting bacterial opsonization and killing. Results in Immunology. 2013;**3**:114-121. DOI: 10.1016/j.rinim.2013.10.004

[44] Barbu EM, Mackenzie C, Foster TJ, Höök M. SdrC induces staphylococcal biofilm formation through a homophilic interaction. Molecular Microbiology. 2014;**1**:172-185. DOI: 10.1111/mmi.12750

[45] Barbu EM, Ganesh VK, Gurusiddappa S, Mackenzie RC, Foster TJ, Sudhof TC, et al. β-Neurexin is a ligand for the *Staphylococcus aureus* MSCRAMM SdrC. PLoS Pathogens. 2010;**1**:e1000726. DOI: 10.1371/journal.ppat.1000726

[46] Sitkiewicz I, Babiak I, Hryniewicz W. Characterization of transcription within sdr region of *Staphylococcus aureus*. Antonie Van Leeuwenhoek. 2011;**2**:409-416. DOI: 10.1007/s10482-010-9476-7

[47] Cheng AG, Kim HK, Burts ML, Krausz T, Schneewind O, Missiakas DM. Genetic requirements for *Staphylococcus aureus* abscess formation and persistence in host tissues. The FASEB Journal. 2009;**10**:3393-3404. DOI: 10.1096/fj.09-135467

[48] Hammers CM, Stanley JR. Desmoglein-1, differentiation, and disease. The Journal of Clinical Investigation. 2013;**4**:1419-1422. DOI: 10.1172/JCI69071

[49] Gaudin CF, Grigg JC, Arrieta AL, Murphy ME. Unique heme-iron coordination by the hemoglobin receptor IsdB of *Staphylococcus aureus*. Biochemistry. 2011;**24**:5443-5452. DOI: 10.1021/bi200369p

[50] Farrand AJ, Reniere ML, Ingmer H, Frees D, Skaar EP. Regulation of host hemoglobin binding by the *Staphylococcus aureus* Clp proteolytic system. Journal of Bacteriology. 2013;**22**:5041-5050. DOI: 10.1128/JB.00505-13

[51] Pishchany G, Dickey SE, Skaar EP. Subcellular localization of the *Staphylococcus aureus* heme iron transport components IsdA and IsdB. Infection and Immunity. 2009;**7**:2624-2634. DOI: 10.1128/IAI.01531-08

[52] Contreras H, Chim N, Credali A, Goulding CW. Heme uptake in bacterial

pathogens. Current Opinion in Chemical Biology. 2014;**19**:34-41. DOI: 10.1016/j.cbpa.2013.12.014

[53] Hammer ND, Skaar EP. Molecular mechanisms of *Staphylococcus aureus* iron acquisition. Annual Review of Microbiology. 2011;**65**:129-147. DOI: 10.1146/annurev-micro-090110-102851

[54] Yoshii Y, Okuda KI, Yamada S, Nagakura M, Sugimoto S, Nagano T, et al. Norgestimate inhibits staphylococcal biofilm formation and resensitizes methicillin-resistant *Staphylococcus aureus* to β-lactam antibiotics. NPJ Biofilms Microbiomes. 2017;**1**:1-9. DOI: 10.1038/s41522-017-0026-1

[55] Yonemoto K, Chiba A, Sugimoto S, Sato C, Saito M, Kinjo Y, et al. Redundant and distinct roles of secreted protein Eap and cell wall-anchored protein SasG in biofilm formation and pathogenicity of *Staphylococcus aureus*. Infection and Immunity. 2019;**4**:e00894-e00818. DOI: 10.1128/IAI.00894-18

[56] Geoghegan JA, Corrigan RM, Gruszka DT, Speziale P, O'Gara JP, Potts JR, et al. Role of surface protein SasG in biofilm formation by *Staphylococcus aureus*. Journal of Bacteriology. 2010;**21**:5663-5673. DOI: 10.1128/JB.00628-10

[57] Formosa-Dague C, Speziale P, Foster TJ, Geoghegan JA, Dufrêne YF. Zinc-dependent mechanical properties of *Staphylococcus aureus* biofilm-forming surface protein SasG. Proceedings of the National Academy of Sciences of the United States of America. 2016;**2**:410-415. DOI: 10.1073/pnas.1519265113

[58] Paharik AE, Horswill AR. The staphylococcal biofilm: Adhesins, regulation, and host response. Microbiology Spectrum. 2016;**2**:529-566. DOI: 10.1128/microbiolspec.VMBF-0022-2015

[59] Sakr A, Brégeon F, Mège JL, Rolain JM, Blin O. *Staphylococcus aureus* nasal colonization: An update on mechanisms, epidemiology, risk factors, and subsequent infections. Frontiers in Microbiology. 2018;**9**:2419. DOI: 10.3389/fmicb.2018.02419

[60] Corrigan RM, Rigby D, Handley P, Foster TJ. The role of *Staphylococcus aureus* surface protein SasG in adherence and biofilm formation. Microbiology. 2007;**8**:2435-2446. DOI: 10.1099/mic.0.2007/006676-0

[61] Crosby HA, Kwiecinski J, Horswill AR. *Staphylococcus aureus* aggregation and coagulation mechanisms, and their function in host–pathogen interactions. Advances in Applied Microbiology. 2016;**96**:1-41. DOI: 10.1016/bs.aambs.2016.07.018

[62] Kwiecinski JM, Crosby HA, Valotteau C, Hippensteel JA, Nayak MK, Chauhan AK, et al. *Staphylococcus aureus* adhesion in endovascular infections is controlled by the ArlRS–MgrA signaling cascade. PLoS Pathogens. 2019;**5**:e1007800. DOI: 10.1371/journal.ppat.1007800

[63] Li M, Du X, Villaruz AE, Diep BA, Wang D, Song Y, et al. MRSA epidemic linked to a quickly spreading colonization and virulence determinant. Nature Medicine. 2012;**5**:816-819. DOI: 10.1038/nm.2692

[64] Otto M. MRSA virulence and spread. Cellular Microbiology. 2012;**10**:1513-1521. DOI: 10.1111/j.1462-5822.2012.01832.x

[65] Nakaminami H, Ito T, Han X, Ito A, Matsuo M, Uehara Y, et al. First report of sasX-positive methicillin-resistant *Staphylococcus aureus* in Japan. FEMS

Microbiology Letters. 2017;**16**:fnx171. DOI: 10.1093/femsle/fnx171

[66] Villanueva San Martín M, García Martínez B, Valle Turrillas J, Rapún Araiz B, Ruiz de los Mozos Aliaga I, Solano Goñi C, et al. Sensory deprivation in *Staphylococcus aureus*. Nature Communications. 2018;**9**:523. DOI: 10.1038/s41467-018-02949-y

[67] Kawada-Matsuo M, Yoshida Y, Nakamura N, Komatsuzawa H. Role of two-component systems in the resistance of *Staphylococcus aureus* to antibacterial agents. Virulence. 2011;**5**:427-430. DOI: 10.4161/viru.2.5.17711

[68] White MJ, Boyd JM, Horswill AR, Nauseef WM. Phosphatidylinositol-specific phospholipase C contributes to survival of *Staphylococcus aureus* USA300 in human blood and neutrophils. Infection and Immunity. 2014;**4**:1559-1571. DOI: 10.1128/IAI.01168-13

[69] Jenul C, Horswill AR. Regulation of *Staphylococcus aureus* virulence. Microbiology Spectrum. 2019;**1**:669-686. DOI: 10.1128/microbiolspec. GPP3-0031-2018

[70] Thoendel M, Horswill AR. Identification of *Staphylococcus aureus* AgrD residues required for autoinducing peptide biosynthesis. The Journal of Biological Chemistry. 2009;**33**:21828-21838. DOI: 10.1074/jbc.M109.031757

[71] Reffuveille F, Josse J, Vallé Q, Gangloff CM, Gangloff SC. *Staphylococcus aureus* biofilms and their impact on the medical field. In: The Rise of Virulence and Antibiotic Resistance in *Staphylococcus aureus*. Vol. 11. 2017. p. 187. DOI: 10.5772/66380

[72] Reuter K, Steinbach A, Helms V. Interfering with bacterial quorum sensing. Perspectives in Medicinal Chemistry. 2016;**8**:1-15. DOI: 10.4137/PMC.S13209

[73] Salam AM. Quave CL, Targeting virulence in *Staphylococcus aureus* by chemical inhibition of the accessory gene regulator system in vivo. mSphere. 2018;**1**:e00500-e00517. DOI: 10.1128/mSphere.00500-17

[74] Wang B, Muir TW. Regulation of virulence in *Staphylococcus aureus*: Molecular mechanisms and remaining puzzles. Cell Chemical Biology. 2016;**2**:214-224. DOI: 10.1016/j.chembiol.2016.01.004

[75] Arciola CR, Campoccia D, Ravaioli S, Montanaro L. Polysaccharide intercellular adhesin in biofilm: Structural and regulatory aspects. Frontiers in Cellular and Infection Microbiology. 2015;**5**:7. DOI: 10.3389/fcimb.2015.00007

[76] Gordon RJ, Lowy FD. Pathogenesis of methicillin-resistant *Staphylococcus aureus* infection. Clinical Infectious Diseases. 2008;**46**(Suppl 5):350-359. DOI: 10.1086/533591

[77] Otto M. *Staphylococcus aureus* toxins. Current Opinion in Microbiology. 2014;**17**:32-37. DOI: 10.1016/j.mib.2013.11.004

[78] Jenul C, Horswill AR. Regulation of *Staphylococcus aureus* virulence. Microbiology Spectrum. 2018;**6**(1):GPP30031-GPP32018. DOI: 10.1128/microbiolspec.GPP3-0031-2018

[79] Priest NK, Rudkin JK, Feil EJ, van den Elsen JMH, Cheung A, Peacock SJ, et al. From genotype to phenotype: Can systems biology be used to predict Staphylococcus aureus virulence? Nature Reviews Microbiology. 2012;**10**(11):791-797. DOI: 10.1038/nrmicro2880

[80] Otto M. Staphylococcal infections: Mechanisms of biofilm maturation and detachment as critical determinants

of pathogenicity. Annual Review of Medicine. 2013;**64**:175-188. DOI: 10.1146/annurev-med-042711-140023

[81] Lerch MF, Schoenfelder SMK, Marincola G, Wencker FDR, Eckart M, Förstner KU, et al. A non-coding RNA from the intercellular adhesion (*ica*) locus of *Staphylococcus epidermidis* controls polysaccharide intercellular adhesion (PIA)-mediated biofilm formation. Molecular Microbiology. 2019;**6**:1571-1591. DOI: 10.1111/mmi.14238

[82] Cue DR, Lei MG, Lee C. Genetic regulation of the intercellular adhesion locus in staphylococci. Frontiers in Cellular and Infection Microbiology. 2012;**2**:38. DOI: 10.3389/fcimb.2012.00038

[83] Beenken KE, Mrak LN, Griffin LM, Zielinska AK, Shaw LN, Rice KC, et al. Epistatic relationships between *sarA* and *agr* in *Staphylococcus aureus* biofilm formation. PLoS One. 2010;**5**:e10790. DOI: 10.1371/journal.pone.0010790

[84] Schwartz K, Syed AK, Stephenson RE, Rickard AH, Boles BR. Functional amyloids composed of phenol soluble modulins stabilize *Staphylococcus aureus* biofilms. PLoS Pathogens. 2012;**6**:e1002744. DOI: 10.1371/journal.ppat.1002744

[85] Taglialegna A, Navarro S, Ventura S, Garnett JA, Matthews S, Penades JR, et al. Staphylococcal bap proteins build amyloid scaffold biofilm matrices in response to environmental signals. PLoS Pathogens. 2016;**6**:e1005711. DOI: 10.1371/journal.ppat.1005711

[86] Blanco LP, Evans ML, Smith DR, Badtke MP, Chapman MR. Diversity, biogenesis and function of microbial amyloids. Trends in Microbiology. 2012;**2**:66-73. DOI: 10.1016/j.tim.2011.11.005

[87] Periasamy S, Joo HS, Duong AC, Bach THL, Tan VY, Chatterjee SS, et al. How *Staphylococcus aureus* biofilms develop their characteristic structure. Proceedings of the National Academy of Sciences of the United States of America. 2012;**4**:1281-1286. DOI: 10.1073/pnas.1115006109

[88] Zapotoczna M, O'Neill E, O'Gara JP. Untangling the diverse and redundant mechanisms of *Staphylococcus aureus* biofilm formation. PLoS Pathogens. 2016;**7**:e1005671. DOI: 10.1371/journal.ppat.1005671

[89] Bautista-Trujillo GU, Solorio-Rivera JL, Rentería-Solórzano I, Carranza-Germán SI, Bustos-Martínez JA, Arteaga-Garibay RI, et al. Performance of culture media useful for the isolation and presumptive identification of *Staphylococcus aureus* from bovine mastitis. Journal of Medical Microbiology. 2013;**63**:369-376. DOI: 10.1099/jmm.0.046284-0

[90] Thomer L, Emolo C, Thammavongsa V, Kim HK, McAdow ME, Yu W, et al. Antibodies against a secreted product of *Staphylococcus aureus* trigger phagocytic killing. The Journal of Experimental Medicine. 2016;**3**:293-301. DOI: 10.1084/jem.20150074

[91] Zapotoczna M, McCarthy H, Rudkin JK, O'Gara JP, O'Neill E. An essential role for coagulase in *Staphylococcus aureus* biofilm development reveals new therapeutic possibilities for device-related infections. The Journal of Infectious Diseases. 2015;**12**:1883-1893. DOI: 10.1093/infdis/jiv319

[92] Archer NK, Mazaitis MJ, Costerton JW, Leid JG, Powers ME, Shirtliff ME. *Staphylococcus aureus* biofilms: Properties, regulation, and roles in human disease. Virulence. 2011;**5**:445-459. DOI: 10.4161/viru.2.5.17724

[93] Lister JL, Horswill AR. *Staphylococcus aureus* biofilms: Recent developments in biofilm dispersal. Frontiers in Cellular and Infection Microbiology. 2014;**4**:178. DOI: 10.3389/fcimb.2014.00178

[94] Boles BR, Thoendel M, Roth AJ, Horswill AR. Identification of genes involved in polysaccharide-independent *Staphylococcus aureus* biofilm formation. PLoS One. 2010;**4**:e10146. DOI: 10.1371/journal.pone.0010146

[95] Neopane P, Nepal HP, Shrestha R, Uehara O, Abiko Y. In vitro biofilm formation by *Staphylococcus aureus* isolated from wounds of hospital-admitted patients and their association with antimicrobial resistance. International Journal of General Medicine. 2018;**11**:25-32. DOI: 10.2147/IJGM.S153268

[96] Miao J, Lin S, Soteyome T, Peters BM, Li Y, Chen H, et al. Biofilm formation of *Staphylococcus aureus* under food heat processing conditions: First report on CML production within biofilm. Scientific Reports. 2019;**9**:1312. DOI: 10.1038/s41598-018-35558-2

[97] Flemming HC, Wingender J. The biofilm matrix. Nature Reviews Microbiology. 2010;**9**:623-633. DOI: 10.1038/nrmicro2415

[98] Das T, Sharma PK, Krom BP, van der Mei HC, Busscher HJ. Role of eDNA on the adhesion forces between *Streptococcus mutans* and substratum surfaces: Influence of ionic strength and substratum hydrophobicity. Langmuir. 2011;**16**:10113-10118. DOI: 10.1021/la202013m

[99] Okshevsky M, Meyer RL. The role of extracellular DNA in the establishment, maintenance and perpetuation of bacterial biofilms. Critical Reviews in Microbiology. 2013;**3**:341-352. DOI: 10.3109/1040841X.2013.841639

[100] Das T, Krom BP, van der Mei HC, Busscher HJ, Sharma PK. DNA-mediated bacterial aggregation is dictated by acid–base interactions. Soft Matter. 2011;**6**:2927-2935. DOI: 10.1039/C0SM01142H

[101] Salgado-Pabón W, Du Y, Hackett KT, Lyons KM, Arvidson CG, Dillard JP. Increased expression of the type IV secretion system in piliated *Neisseria gonorrhoeae* variants. Journal of Bacteriology. 2010;**7**:1912-1920. DOI: 10.1128/JB.01357-09

[102] DeFrancesco AS, Masloboeva N, Syed AK, DeLoughery A, Bradshaw N, Li GW, et al. Genome-wide screen for genes involved in eDNA release during biofilm formation by *Staphylococcus aureus*. Proceedings of the National Academy of Sciences of the United States of America. 2017;**29**:5969-5978. DOI: 10.1073/pnas.1704544114

[103] Foulston L, Elsholz AK, DeFrancesco AS, Losick R. The extracellular matrix of *Staphylococcus aureus* biofilms comprises cytoplasmic proteins that associate with the cell surface in response to decreasing pH. mBio. 2014;**5**:e01667-e01614. DOI: 10.1128/mBio.01667-14

[104] Dengler V, Foulston L, DeFrancesco AS, Losick R. An electrostatic net model for the role of extracellular DNA in biofilm formation by *Staphylococcus aureus*. Journal of

Bacteriology. 2015;**24**:3779-3787. DOI: 10.1128/JB.00726-15

[105] Kiedrowski MR, Crosby HA, Hernandez FJ, Malone CL, McNamara JO. *Staphylococcus aureus* Nuc2 is a functional, surface-attached extracellular nuclease. PLoS One. 2014;**4**:e95574. DOI: 10.1371/journal.pone.0095574

[106] Moormeier DE, Endres JL, Mann EE, Sadykov MR, Horswill AR, Rice KC, et al. Use of microfluidic technology to analyze gene expression during *Staphylococcus aureus* biofilm formation reveals distinct physiological niches. Applied and Environmental Microbiology. 2013;**11**:3413-3424. DOI: 10.1128/AEM.00395-13

[107] Boles BR, Horswill AR. Staphylococcal biofilm disassembly. Trends in Microbiology. 2011;**9**:449-455. DOI: 10.1016/j.tim.2011.06.004

[108] Houston P, Rowe SE, Pozzi C, Waters EM, O'Gara JP. Essential role for the major autolysin in the fibronectin-binding protein-mediated *Staphylococcus aureus* biofilm phenotype. Infection and Immunity. 2011;**3**:1153-1165. DOI: 10.1128/IAI.00364-10

[109] Sugimoto S, Sato F, Miyakawa R, Chiba A, Onodera S, Hori S, et al. Broad impact of extracellular DNA on biofilm formation by clinically isolated methicillin-resistant and-sensitive strains of *Staphylococcus aureus*. Scientific Reports. 2018;**1**:1-11. DOI: 10.1038/s41598-018-20485-z

[110] Kiedrowski MR, Kavanaugh JS, Malone CL, Mootz JM, Voyich JM, Smeltzer MS, et al. Nuclease modulates biofilm formation in community-associated methicillin-resistant *Staphylococcus aureus*. PLoS One. 2011;**11**:e26714. DOI: 10.1371/journal.pone.0026714

[111] Scherr TD, Hanke ML, Huang O, James DB, Horswill AR, Bayles KW, et al. *Staphylococcus aureus* biofilms induce macrophage dysfunction through leukocidin AB and alpha-toxin. mBio. 2015;**4**:e01021-e01015. DOI: 10.1128/mBio.01021-15

[112] Dastgheyb SS, Villaruz AE, Le KY, Tan VY, Duong AC, Chatterjee SS, et al. Role of phenol-soluble modulins in formation of *Staphylococcus aureus* biofilms in synovial fluid. Infection and Immunity. 2015;**7**:2966-2975. DOI: 10.1128/IAI.00394-15

[113] Oliveira D, Borges A, Simões M. *Staphylococcus aureus* toxins and their molecular activity in infectious diseases. Toxins. 2018;**6**:252. DOI: 10.3390/toxins10060252

Section 3

Diagnosis

Chapter 5

Recent Progress in the Diagnosis of *Staphylococcus* in Clinical Settings

Xue-Di Zhang, Bin Gu, Muhammad Usman, Jia-Wei Tang, Zheng-Kang Li, Xin-Qiang Zhang, Jia-Wei Yan and Liang Wang

Abstract

Staphylococci are mainly found on the skin or in the nose. These bacteria are typically friendly, causing no harm to healthy individuals or resulting in only minor issues that can go away on their own. However, under certain circumstances, staphylococcal bacteria could invade the bloodstream, affect the entire body, and lead to life-threatening problems like septic shock. In addition, antibiotic-resistant *Staphylococcus* is another issue because of its difficulty in the treatment of infections, such as the notorious methicillin-resistant *Staphylococcus aureus* (MRSA) which is resistant to most of the currently known antibiotics. Therefore, rapid and accurate diagnosis of *Staphylococcus* and characterization of the antibiotic resistance profiles are essential in clinical settings for efficient prevention, control, and treatment of the bacteria. This chapter highlights recent advances in the diagnosis of *Staphylococci* in clinical settings with a focus on the advanced technique of surface-enhanced Raman spectroscopy (SERS), which will provide a framework for the real-world applications of novel diagnostic techniques in medical laboratories via bench-top instruments and at the bedside through point-of-care devices.

Keywords: *Staphylococcus*, rapid diagnosis, mass spectrometry, Raman spectrometry, machine-learning algorithm

1. Introduction

Bacteria belonging to the genus *Staphylococcus* is widely distributed in nature and is a common pathogen that causes nosocomial and community-acquired infections. It is a facultatively anaerobic Gram-positive coccus that provides a serious threat to human health due to a combination of toxin-mediated virulence, invasiveness, and antibiotic resistance. *Staphylococcus* is commonly found in the air, water, dust, and human and animal excretions. Every year, Staphylococcus *aureus* (*S. aureus*) causes almost half a million hospitalizations and 50,000 deaths in the United States [1]. This chapter reviewed the recent progress in the diagnosis of staphylococcal bacteria in clinical settings, including the variety of commonly used techniques ranging from traditional culture to emerging molecular methods. Conventionally, the accurate identification of clinical isolates of *Staphylococcus* needs a battery of tests, which is costly in resource-limited settings, though biochemical tests and drug susceptibility methods have the advantages of low cost and easy operation. However, these methods are limited to phenotypic detection only. The nucleic acid amplification methods such as PCR, real-time fluorescence quantification of nucleic acids and ring-mediated isothermal amplification are sensitive and can detect genes for strain typing. In addition, new technologies such as matrix-assisted laser desorption ionization time-of-flight mass spectrometry, gene sequencing, and SERS are ideal for phenotypic abnormalities, slow growth, and culture-negative infections, etc. The principles, characteristics, and applications of which are therefore reviewed, with an emphasis on the use of SERS as an emerging technique for the detection of bacterial pathogens more efficiently.

2. Clinical significance of *Staphylococcus* infections

2.1 Staphylococcal species

The genus *Staphylococcus* belongs to a diverse group of Micrococcaceae bacteria that can cause many diseases. They have the capacity to produce a wide range of extracellular toxins and cell surface virulence factors. There are currently 85 species and 30 subspecies in the genus [2]. Although most people have antibodies with bodies to staphylococcal infection, these are usually ineffective, and the disease can reoccur multiple times [3] . *Staphylococci* can cause a variety of infections: (1) *S. aureus* causes localized abscesses in different places and superficial skin diseases (boils, styes) [4]; (2) *S. aureus* causes deep-seated infections like osteomyelitis, endocarditis, and potentially fatal skin infections [5]; (3) *S. aureus*, along with *Staphylococcus epidermidis*, is a leading cause of hospital-acquired (nosocomial) surgical wound infection and infections caused by indwelling medical device [6]; (4) *S. aureus* releases enterotoxins into food, which causes food poisoning [7]; (5) *S. aureus* releases superantigens into the bloodstream, which results in toxic shock syndrome [8]; and (6) urinary tract infections are caused by *Staphylococcus saprophyticus*, particularly in females [9]. Other *Staphylococci* species, e.g., *Staphylococcus lugdunensis*, *Staphylococcus haemolyticus*, *Staphylococcus warneri*, *Staphylococcus schleiferi*, and *S. intermedius*, are uncommon pathogens. *Staphylococcus* parasites in humans and primates mainly include the following: *S.* aureus, *S. epidermidis*, *Staphylococcus capitis*, *Staphylococcus caprae*, *S. saccharolyticus, S. warneri, S. haemolyticus, Staphylococcus hominis, S. saprophyticus, Staphylococcus pasteuri,* and *Staphylococcus xylosus,* etc., among which *S. aureus* colonizes the nasal canals, axillae, and pharynx [10–12], while *S. epidermidis* is a widespread human skin commensal [13]. In addition, *Staphylococcus* species are usually divided into coagulase-positive *Staphylococcus* (CPS) represented by *S. aureus,* and coagulase-negative *Staphylococcus* (CNS) represented by *S. epidermidis*. The most common type *is S. aureus subsp. aureus,* among the clonal populations followed by *S. epidermidis*, *S. haemolyticus*, and *S. saprophyticus subsp. saprophyticus*, etc.

2.2 Staphylococcal biological properties

Staphylococcus is spherical or oval in shape, 0.5–1.5 μm in diameter, forming single, paired, quadruple, short-chain, and irregular grape bunches or clusters. *Staphylococcus* has no flagella and no spores except for a few strains which generally do not form capsules [14]. *S. aureus* produces a wide range of extracellular proteins and polysaccharides, a number of which are associated with virulence [15]. Except for *S. aureus subsp. anaerobius* and *S. saccharolyticus*, most *Staphylococci* are facultative anaerobes. The nutritional requirements for cultivation are not stringent, and the optimum pH is 7.4–7.6.

Staphylococcus can grow well on blood agar, brain heart infusion agar, tryptone soy agar, and mannitol salt agar [16]. After 24 h of incubation in the atmospheric environment at 34–37°C, they can form round, smooth, neat-edged, raised, moist, opaque, creamy, porcelain white, pale yellow, or orange-yellow colonies. *S. aureus subsp. anaerobius*, *S. saccharolyticus*, *Staphylococcus auricularis*, *Staphylococcus vitulinus*, *S. lentus*, and *Staphylococcus equorum* grow slowly and gradually, and their colonies are commonly seen after 36 h of incubation. Small colony variants (SCVs) of *Staphylococcus* grow extremely slowly on conventional medium and the colony color is lighter with less pigment [17]. *Staphylococci* are generally salt-tolerant and grow well on agar with 6.5% NaCl. Some Staphylococcal species like *S. aureus* can produce hemolysin, and an apparent β-hemolytic ring can be seen after 24 h of incubation on sheep blood or rabbit blood agar [18]. When routinely cultured, many *Staphylococci* produce fat-soluble carotenoids visible to the naked eye, making the colonies yellow, orange-yellow, or orange and not spread into the agar medium. *Staphylococcus* does not form pigment in liquid medium, grows uniformly and turbidly, slightly precipitates at the bottom of the tube, and is easy to disperse when shaken. *S. aureus* colonies are yellow on Mannitol Salt Medium (MSM). White precipitation rings can be formed around *S. aureus* colonies on Egg-Yolk Salt Agar Medium. Moreover, *S. aureus* colonies are black on Baird-Parker agar, surrounded by turbid bands and transparent rings. The surface antigens of *Staphylococcus* are mainly *Staphylococcus* Protein A (SPA) and polysaccharide antigens. SPA is a surface protein on the cell wall with species and genus specificity while polysaccharide antigens are type-specific. *Staphylococcus* is one of the most resistant non-spore-forming bacteria, which is resistant to dryness and high salinity and can grow in a medium containing 100–150 g/l NaCl.

2.3 Distribution and epidemiology

Staphylococcus is widely distributed in nature, mainly parasitic on mammals and birds' skin, sebaceous glands and mucous membranes. Some *Staphylococcus* and its subspecies are parasitic in selected parts of the host. *S. capitis subsp. capitis* mainly exists in great amounts in the sebaceous glands on the top of the head and forehead of humans, while *S. capitis subsp. ureolyticus* is present in abundance in the armpits of humans. *S. aureus* has the dual characteristics of a colonized and pathogenic bacterium, mainly distributed in the nasal vestibule. About 20% of people have persistent nasal cavity colonization by *S. aureus*, and 30% have intermittent colonization. In addition, *S. aureus* is also colonized in the axilla, pharynx, groin and gastrointestinal tract, etc. [13]. It has been shown in the study that *S. aureus* strains isolated from the blood of 82% of patients with bacteremia are identical to those isolated from the nasal cavity [3, 19]. More than 50 million people are expected to be infected with methicillin-resistant *S. aureus* (MRSA), which is easily transmitted through skin contact. However, MRSA infection is difficult to cure due to its resistance to most antibiotics, while children, elderly people, and sick patients in hospitals and nursing homes are particularly susceptible. While the number of MRSA bloodstream infections in the US has declined in recent years, the infection still resulted in 20,000 fatalities in 2017. In addition, MRSA was responsible for more than 100,000 deaths worldwide in 2019, highlighting the importance of improved surveillance to prevent and manage the spread of this potentially dangerous bacterium [20]. *S. epidermidis* is the most common *Staphylococcus* on the human body surface, especially in moist areas such as armpits, groin, perineum, anterior nostrils, and toes [21]. *S. haemolyticus* is easily isolated from the apocrine glands in the axilla [16]. In addition, *S. saprophyticus subsp. saprophyticus* is easily isolated from the female rectum and urinary system [22].

2.4 Staphylococcal infections

S. aureus bacteremia, which often leads to metastatic foci of infection, can occur at any site, but it is especially common with infections associated with intravascular catheters. *S. epidermidis* and other coagulase-negative *Staphylococci* are gradually causing hospital-acquired bacteremia because they can form biofilms on intravascular catheters and other foreign objects. *Staphylococcal* bacteremia is a substantial reason for disease and death in debilitated people [23]. Many *Staphylococci* are opportunistic pathogens of the skin and mucous membranes. *S. aureus* is the primary clinic pathogenic bacteria of humans [24]. The diseases caused by the bacterium can be roughly divided into purulent infections and toxin-causing diseases. The former includes superficial infections (boils, carbuncles, folliculitis, paronychia, styes, wound suppuration, abscesses), deep tissue infections (mastitis, cellulitis, necrotizing fasciitis, osteomyelitis, arthritis), and systemic infections like bacteremia. Toxin-related diseases caused by *S. aureus* mainly include staphylococcal scalded skin syndrome (SSSS) caused by an exfoliative toxin, also known as exfoliative dermatitis; toxic shock syndrome (TSS) caused by toxic shock syndrome toxin-1 (TSST-1) and *S. aureus* food poisoning (SFP) caused by staphylococcal enterotoxins (SEs). Lymphangitis is caused by bacterial infection of the lymphatic vessels. The organisms that cause the disease enter the body through a skin wound and are either *Streptococcus* or *Staphylococcus*. The inflamed lymph vessels appear as red streaks under the skin that extend from the infection site to the groin or armpit. The other symptoms may include fever, chills, headache, and appetite loss. The most typical manifestation of staphylococcal disease is skin infections. Superficial infections can be generalized with vesicular pustules and crusting (impetigo) or focal with nodular abscesses (furuncles and carbuncles). Deeper cutaneous abscesses are relatively common. There could be severe necrotizing skin infections. Staphylococcal newborn infections, which can cause skin lesions with or without exfoliation, bacteremia, meningitis, and pneumonia, typically appear within 6 weeks of delivery [25].

Coagulase-negative staphylococci (CNS) represented by *S. epidermidis* have become the leading pathogen of nosocomial infection in recent years. They can cause prosthetic valve endocarditis, urinary system infection, central nervous system infection, and bacteremia. *S. lugdunensis* can cause endocarditis, arthritis, urinary tract infections and bacteremia. In addition, *S. saprophyticus* can often cause urinary tract infection, prostatitis, wound infections, bacteremia, and so on. Chronic infection or intracellular parasitism of *S. aureus* often appears in the form of SCVs during in vitro culture [26]. SCVs are now defined as a subgroup of microorganisms that grow slowly on agar medium, form small colonies, have reduced or absent pigment production, and have altered expression of virulence factors (e.g., reduced production of α-hemolysin). This is quite different from typical *S. aureus* colonies, so it is easy to miss its detection in routine microbial identification. However, SCVs are closely related to chronic and recurrent infections [27, 28]. Typical *S. aureus* colonies and SCVs often coexist on agar medium. Therefore, in-depth study of SCVs is critical to the treatment and control of clinical infections.

3. Traditional identification of staphylococcal bacteria

3.1 Microscopic inspection and culture

Microscopic inspection is based on performing morphological tests on colonies. Clinical specimens were smeared, Gram-stained, and the morphology was observed under a microscope. *S. aureus* is typically identified using tests for clumping factor, coagulase, hemolysins, and thermostable deoxyribonuclease. There are currently available latex agglutination tests. The identity of *S. epidermidis* is established by using commercial bio-typing kits. *Staphylococci* are catalase positive and can withstand quite high sodium chloride concentrations (7.5–10%). This feature is often used in the preparation of *Staphylococci*-specific media. A rapid and efficient method for classifying Gram-positive bacteria species was developed using hyperspectral microscope images. Traditional bacteria detection and identification procedures using specific agar media remain the "gold standard" to differentiate the microorganisms. Furthermore, traditional serotyping approaches based on antibodies or genetic matching, such as plasmid fingerprinting, have been developed [29].

3.2 Staphylococcal biochemical identification

The majority of staphylococcal oxidase tests are negative. *Staphylococcus sciuri*, *S. vitulinus*, *S. lentus*, *Staphylococcus fleurettii,* and *Staphylococcus caseolyticus* are positive for oxidase tests due to the presence of Cytochrome c oxidase. *Staphylococcus* catalase tests are usually positive, while *S. aureus subsp. anaerobius* and *S. saccharolyticus* are negative. Most *Staphylococcus* species can decompose a variety of carbohydrates and deoxidize nitrates, as they are sensitive to lysostaphin and furazolidone, and are resistant to bacitracin and vibriostatic agent O/129 (2,4-diamino-6,7-diisopropylpteridine). The plasma coagulase test and the thermostable nuclease test for *S. aureus* are positive. *S. aureus* is sensitive to novobiocin. The biochemical identification of *Staphylococcus* and other Gram-positive cocci is shown in **Table 1**. It can be known from the table that *Staphylococcus* catalase is positive, which is different from *Enterococcus* and *Streptococcus*. The identification of biochemical reactions within the *Staphylococcus* species is shown in **Table 2**. Mature commercial biochemical identification systems include API Staph (bioMérieux), ID32 Staph (bioMérieux), Vitek (bioMérieux), MicroScan Product Pos ID family (Siemens Health-care Diagnostics), BD BBL Crystal (BD Diagnostics Systems), Sensitire GPID (TREK Diagnostic Systems), etc. Most laboratories use commercial identification systems or automated identification instruments. These methods are simple, convenient, and accurate. However, uncommon strains or strains with phenotypic variants (such as SCVs) require molecular identification due to altered biochemical response patterns.

3.3 Antibiotic resistance

The conventional approaches for antibiotic susceptibility testing of *Staphylococci* include disk diffusion and broth dilution, which can be operated following the American Clinical and Laboratory Standards Institute (CLSI) and the European Committee for Antimicrobial Susceptibility Testing (EUCAST). The disc diffusion method, also known as the Kirby-Bauer (K-B) method, is based on the principle of sticking a disc containing anti-bacteial drugs onto an agar plate inoculated with the test bacteria. The medicine in the disc absorbs the water in the agar and dissolves continuously to spread around

Characteristic	*Staphylococcus*	*Micrococcus*	*Enterococcus*	*Balloon fungus*	*Megacoccus*	*Streptococcus*	*Kineococcus*
Colony pigment	White/yellow	Yellow/milk white	White/yellow	White	White	Colorless/gray	ND
G + C(%)	30–39	66–75	34–42	35–40	38–45	34–46	39–52
Strictly aerobic	–	+	–	–	±	–	+
Quadruple arrangement	d	+	–	+	d	–	+
Motility	–	–	d	–	–	–	+
6.5% NaCl	+	+	+	+	+	d	+
Catalase	+	+	–	–	+	–	+
Oxidase (modified method)	–	+	–	–	+	–	ND
Glucose anaerobic acid production	d	–	+	(±)	–	+	–
Glycerol aerobic acid production	+	–	d	ND	ND	d	–
Benzidine test	+	+	–	–	ND	–	+
Erythromycin (0.4 ug/ml)	R	S	R	ND	R	S	ND
Bacitracin (0.04 U/disk)	R	S	R	S	R	d	ND
Furazolidone (100 ug/disk)	S	R	S	S	S	S	S
Glucolysin (200 ug/disk)	S	R	R	R	R	R	R

Note: Abbreviations: +, more than 90% of the strains are positive; ±, more than 90% of the strains are weakly positive; –, more than 90% of the strains are negative; d, 11–89% of the strains are positive; ND, uncertain; (+–), Delayed response; S, sensitive; R, resistant.

Table 1.
Main biochemical identifications of Staphylococcus and other gram-positive cocci.

Species	**Colony size**	**Colony Pigment**	**Anaerobic growth**	**aerobic growth**	**Hemolysis**	**Coagulase**	**Agglutination factor**	**Catalase**	**Oxidase**	**Thermo-nuclease**	**ALP**	**PRY**
S. aureus subsp. aureus	+	+	+	+	+	+	+	+	–	+	+	–
S. aureus subsp. anaerobius	–	–	(+)	(+)	+	+	–	–	–	+	+	ND
Staphylococcus hyicus	+	–	+	+	–	d	–	+	–	+	+	–
S. intermedius	+	–	(+)	+	d	+	d	+	–	+	+	+
Staphylococcus lugdunensis	d	d	+	+	(+)	–	(+)	+	–	–	–	+
Staphylococcus schleiferi subsp. coagulans	–	–	+	+	(+)	–	+	+	–	+	+	+
S. schleiferi subsp. schleiferi	d	–	+	+	(+)	+	–	+	–	+	+	ND
Staphylococcus delphini	+	–	(+)	+	+	+	–	+	–	–	+	ND
S. hutrae	–	–	+	+	+	+	–	+	–	(±)	+	ND
Staphylococcus sciuri subsp. carnaticus	–	d	(d)	+	(±)	–	d	+	+	–	d	–
S. sciuri subsp. rodentium	d	d	(d)	+	(±)	–	+	+	+	–	d	–
Staphylococcus pseudintermedius	+	–	ND	+	+	+	–	+	ND	+	+	+
Staphylococcus epidermidis	–	–	+	+	(d)	–	–	+	–	–	+	–

Species	ODC	Urease	Arginine utilization	Nitrate reduction	V-P	Aescin hydrolysis	Galactosidase	Novobiocin resistance	Polymyxin B resistance	α-Lactose	Maltose	Sucrose
S. aureus subsp. aureus	–	d	+	+	+	–	–	–	+	+	+	+
S. aureus subsp. anaerobius	ND	ND	ND	–	–	––	–	–	ND	–	+	+
Staphylococcus hyicus	–	d	+	+	–	–	–	–	+	+	–	+
S. intermedius	–	+	d	+	–	–	+	–	–	d	(±)	+
Staphylococcus lugdunensis	+	d	–	+	+	–	–	–	d	+	+	+
Staphylococcus schleiferi subsp. coagulans	–	–	+	+	+	–	(+)	–	–	–	–	–
S. schleiferi subsp. schleiferi	ND	+	+	+	+	ND	ND	–	ND	d	–	d
Staphylococcus delphini	ND	+	+	+	–	ND	ND	–	ND	+	+	+
S. hutrae	ND	+	–	+	–	ND	+	–	ND	+	+	ND
Staphylococcus sciuri subsp. carnaticus	–	–	–	+	–	+	–	+	–	(d)	(d)	+
S. sciuri subsp. rodentium	–	–	–	+	–	+	–	+	–	(d)	(d)	+
Staphylococcus pseudintermedius	ND	+	ND	+	ND	ND	+	–	ND	+	+	+
Staphylococcus epidermidis	(d)	+	d	+	+	–	–	–	+	d	+	+

Species	Colony size	Colony Pigment	Anaerobic growth	aerobic growth	Hemolysis	Coagulase	Agglutination factor	Catalase	Oxidase	Thermonuclease	ALP	PRY
Staphylococcus haemolyticus	+	d	(+)	+	(+)	–	–	+	–	–	–	+
Staphylococcus saprophyticus subsp. saprophyticus	+	d	(+)	+	–	–	–	+	–	–	–	+
S. saprophyticus subsp. bovis	–	+	+	+	–	–	–	+	–	–	–	–
Staphylococcus warneri	d	d	+	+	(d)	–	–	+	–	–	–	–
Staphylococcus hominis subsp. hominis	–	d	–	+	–	–	–	+	–	–	–	–
S. hominis subsp. novobiosepticus	–	–	–	+	–	–	–	+	–	–	–	+
S. simulans	+	–	+	+	(d)	–	–	+	–	–	(d)	+
Staphylococcus capitis subsp. capitis	–	–	(+)	+	(d)	–	–	+	–	–	–	–
S. capitis subsp. ureolyticus	–	(d)	(+)	+	(d)	–	–	+	–	–	–	(d)
Staphylococcus cohnii subsp. cohnii	d	–	d	+	(d)	–	–	+	–	–	–	–
S. cohnii subsp. urealyticus	+	d	(+)	+	(d)	–	–	+	–	–	+	d
Staphylococcus xylosus	+	d	d	+	–	–	–	+	–	–	d	d

Staphylococcus caprae	d	–	(+)	+	(d)	–	–	+	–	–	(+)	d

Species	ODC	Urease	Arginine utilization	Nitrate reduction	V-P	Aescin hydrolysis	Galactosidase	Novobiocin resistance	Polymyxin B resistance	α-Lactose	Maltose	Sucrose
Staphylococcus haemolyticus	–	–	+	+	+	–	–	–	–	d	+	+
Staphylococcus saprophyticus subsp. saprophyticus	–	+	–	–	+	–	+	+	–	d	+	+
S. saprophyticus subsp. bovis	–	+	–	+	d	–	d	+	ND	–	+	+
Staphylococcus warneri	–	+	d	d	+	–	–	–	–	d	(+)	+
Staphylococcus hominis subsp. hominis	–	+	d	d	d	–	–	–	–	d	+	(+)
S. hominis subsp. novobiosepticus	–	+	–	d	d	+	–	+	ND	d	+	(+)
S. simulans	–	+	+	+	d	–	+	–	d	+	(±)	+
Staphylococcus capitis subsp. capitis	–	–	d	d	d	–	–	–	–	(+)	–	(+)
S. capitis subsp. ureolyticus	–	+	+	+	d	–	–	–	ND	+	+	+
Staphylococcus cohnii subsp. cohnii	–	–	–	–	d	–	–	+	–	–	(d)	–
S. cohnii subsp. urealyticus	–	+	–	–	d	–	+	+	–	+	(+)	–

DOI: http://dx.doi.org/10.5772/intechopen.108524

Staphylococcus xylosus	−	+	−	d	d	d	+	+	−	d	+	+
Staphylococcus caprae	−	+	+	+	+	−	−	−	−	+	(d)	−

Notes: Abbreviations: +, more than 90% of strains are positive; ±, above 90% of strains are weakly positive; −, above 90% of strains are negative; d, 11–89% of positive strains; ND, uncertain; (+−), delayed response. ALP stands for alkaline phosphatase; PRY stands for pyrrolidone amino amidase test; and ODC stands for ornithine decarboxylase.

Table 2.
Identification of biochemical reactions within the species of Staphylococcus.

Species	Resistant phenotype	Test method	Medium	Drug	Incubation conditions	Results	Quality control	Whether or not to be confirmed
S. aureus	Oxacillin Resistance[a]	Oxacillin-Salt Agar Screen	MHA + 4%NaCl	6 ug/ml Oxacillin	33–35°C, ambient air, 24 h	≥1 colony	S. aureus ATCC®29213 S. aureus ATCC® 43300	No
	mecA-Mediated Oxacillin Resistance[a]	Cefoxitin Broth Microdilution	CAMHB	Cefoxitin	33–35°C, ambient air, 16–20 h	>4 ug/ml = *mecA* Positive, ≤4 ug/ml = *mecA* negative	S. aureus ATCC®25,923	No
		Cefoxitin Disk Diffusion	MHA	30 μg Cefoxitin disk	35± 2 °C, ambient air, 16–18 h	≤21 mm = *mecA* Positive, ≥22 mm = *mecA* negative	S. aureus ATCC®25,923	No
	Vancomycin MIC ≥ 8 ug/ml	BHI agar dilution	BHI agar	6 ug/ml Vancomycin	35 ± 2 °C, aerobic, 24 h	≥1 colony, presumptive susceptibility reduced	Enterococcus faecalis ATCC® 29,212	Yes
		Disc Diffusion	MHA	30 ug Vancomycin disk	35 ± 2°C, 16–18 h	6 mm, presumptive resistant	S. aureus ATCC®25,923	Yes
	Inducible Clindamycin Resistance	Clindamycin-Erythromycin Broth Microdilution	CAMHB	4 ug Erythromycin and 0.5 ug Clindamycin in the same well	35 ± 2 °C,ambient air, 18–24 h	Any growth = positive, no growth = non-inducible clindamycin resistance	S. aureus ATCC®BAA-976, S. aureus ATCC®BAA-977	No
		D test (Disc Diffusion)	MHA or BAP	15 ug Erythromycin disk and 2 fug Clindamycin disk are placed 15–26 mm apart	35 ± 2 °C, ambient air, 16–18 h	zone edge appears "truncated" (similar to the English letter D) = positive; blurred zone edge (beach-like) = Clindamycin resistance	S. aureus ATCC®BAA-976, S. aureus ATCC®BAA-977	No
	High-Level Mupirocin Resistance	Broth Microdilution	CAMHB	256 ug/ml Mupirocin	35 ± 2°C, ambient air, 24 h	grow = *mup A*positive	S. aureus ATCC®29,213, S. aureus ATCC®BAA-1708	No

Species	Resistant phenotype	Test method	Medium	Drug	Incubation conditions	Results	Quality control	Whether or not to be confirmed
		Disc Diffusion	MHA	200 ug Mupirocin disk	35 ± 2 °C, ambient air, 24 h	no inhibition zone = *mupA* positive, any inhibition zone = *mupA negative*	S. aureus ATCC®25,923, S. aureus ATCC®BAA-1708	No
CoNS	*mecA-Mediated Oxacillin Resistance*[b]	Cefoxitin Disk Diffusion	MHA	30 μg Cefoxitin disk	33–35°C, ambient air, 24 h	≤24 mm = *mecA*Positive, ≥25 mm = *mecA* negative	S. aureus ATCC® 43,300	No
	Inducible Clindamycin Resistance	Clindamycin-Erythromycin Broth Microdilution	CAMHB	4 ug Erythromycin and 0.5 ug Clindamycin in the same well	35 ± 2 °C, ambient air, 18–24 h	Any growth = positive, no growth = non-inducible clindamycin resistance	S. aureus ATCC®BAA-976, S. aureus ATCC®BAA-977	No
	β-Lactamase Production	Disk diffusion (Penicillin zone-edge test)	MHA	10 units penicillin disk	35 ± 2 °C, ambient air, 16–20 h	Sharp zone edge = *β-Lactamase* positive, blurred zone edge = β-Lactamase negative	S. aureus ATCC®25,923	No
		Nitrocefin-based test	N/A	N/A	<1 h or according to the manufacturer's instructions for use	From yellow to red or pink = β-lactamase positive	S. aureus ATCC®29,213 S. aureus ATCC® 25,923	Yes
		D test (Disc Diffusion)	MHA or BAP	15 ug Erythromycin disk and 2 ug Clindamycin disk are placed 15–26 mm apart	35 ± 2 °C, ambient air, 16–18 h	zone edge appears "truncated" (similar to the English letter D) = positive; blurred zone edge (beach-like) = clindamycin resistance	S. aureus ATCC®BAA-976, S. aureus ATCC®BAA-977	No

Species	Resistant phenotype	Test method	Medium	Drug	Incubation conditions	Results	Quality control	Whether or not to be confirmed
	β-lactamase production	Nitrocefin-based test	N/A	N/A	<1 h or according to the manufacturer's instructions for use	From yellow to red or pink = β-lactamase positive	S. aureus ATCC®29,213 S. aureus ATCC® 25,923	Yes

[a]*For S. aureus and S. lugdunensis, although S. lugdunensis is a CNS, some resistant phenotypes are more consistent with S. aureus.*
[b]*For CoNS, except for S. lugdunensis and Staphylococcus pseudintermedius.*
Note: Abbreviations: BHI, brain heart infusion; CAMHB, calcium-adjusted MH broth; MHA, MH agar plate; BAP, blood plate; ATCC, American Type Culture Collection.

Table 3.
The main resistant phenotypes and screening methods of Staphylococcus.

the disc. The growth of bacteria is inhibited within the range of inhibitory concentration around the disc, thus forming a transparent antibacterial ring. Its size reflects the susceptibility of the test bacteria to the drug and is negatively correlated with the test bacteria's minimum inhibitory concentration (MIC). The principle of the broth dilution method is to use Mueller Hinton Broth (MHB) to dilute the antibacterial drugs to different concentrations and then culture the bacteria. The MIC or the minimal bactericidal concentration (MBC) is tested by observing the growth of the bacteria.

Commercial detection systems for the broth dilution method for drug susceptibility mainly include bioMérieux (http://www.biomerieuxusa.com), Siemens Healthcare Diagnostics (http://www.siemens.com), Becton Dickinson Diagnostics (http://www.bd.com) and Thermo Scientific (http://www.thermoscientific.com). *S. aureus* and *S. epidermidis* have no natural resistance, while *S. saprophyticus*, *Staphylococcus cohnii*, and *S. xylosus* are naturally resistant to novobiocin, and *S. saprophyticus* and *Staphylococcus kloosii* are naturally resistant to fosfomycin. The common resistant phenotypes and screening methods of *Staphylococcus* are shown in **Table 3**. *S. aureus* is a serious danger to worldwide public health security, especially methicillin-resistant *S. aureus* (MRSA), which has become the leading pathogen of nosocomial infections worldwide. Besides that, drug-resistant genes of multidrug-resistant *S. aureus* strains can be spread among humans, animals, and the environment through horizontal transfer [30], making the problem of bacterial drug resistance increasingly serious. Turner et al. [31] reported that *S. aureus* had developed different degrees of resistance to almost all antibiotics in the past 10 years. MRSA refers to *S. aureus* carrying the *mecA* gene and (or) *S. aureus* with a MIC of Oxacillin >4 mg/l, which can be divided into hospital-acquired (HA-MRSA) and community-acquired (CA-MRSA) strains. The drug resistance mechanism of MASA is complex and mainly related to the *mecA* gene encoding penicillin-binding protein PBP2a [32], the *mecC* gene encoding penicillin-binding protein PBP2c [33, 34], exogenous acquisition of staphylococcal chromosome *mec* gene [35], *fem* gene [36, 37] and other factors.

The cefoxitin disk diffusion assay of *mecA*-mediated oxacillin resistance for CoNS in **Table 3** does not apply to *S. lugdunensis* and *S. pseudintermedius*. The detection method of *S. lugdunensis* is the same as that of *S. aureus*. The oxacillin resistance of *S. pseudintermedius* was detected by 1 μg oxacillin disk, while the cefoxitin disc and the MIC methods were both unreliable. When using vancomycin to treat *S. aureus*, *S. aureus* is easy to develop from sensitivity to an intermediate or resistance phenotype. Attention should be paid to the detection of vancomycin sensitivity to *S. aureus*. The detection of vancomycin-intermediate *S. aureus* (VISA) and vancomycin-resistant *S. aureus* (VRSA) by automated drug susceptibility systems or disc diffusion methods is complex and the results are unreliable. Therefore, further confirmation is required. Biochemical identification and routine drug susceptibility testing require the acquisition of pure cultured colonies, which is time-consuming for slow-growing staphylococci.

4. Rapid diagnosis of Staphylococcal infections

4.1 PCR and its derived technologies

4.1.1 Polymerase chain reaction (PCR)

Polymerase chain reaction (PCR) is the most extensively used nucleic acid amplification method for bacterial serotyping and confirmation. RT-PCR (Real-time quantitative

PCR) has high sensitivity, high specificity, low pollution, and a high degree of automation [38]. Its reaction is monitored in real-time and can quantitatively detect target genes. The detection time of clinical samples can even be shortened to 1 h. Recent literature reports show that RT-PCR technology is currently the most accurate, reproducible and internationally recognized standard method for the quantitative and qualitative detection of nucleic acid molecules. For example, Okolie et al. [39] simultaneously detected marker genes of Coagulase-negative *Staphylococcus* (CoNS), staphylococcal protein A (SPA), Panton-Valentine leukocidin (PVL) and methicillin-resistant *S. aureus* (MRSA) by applying real-time PCR polymorphism analysis. Yang et al. [40] also found that the effect of real-time RT-PCR in detecting methicillin-resistant *S. aureus* (MRSA) was better than drug susceptibility testing. The enterotoxin produced by *S. aureus* in food can cause food poisoning, so *S. aureus* is also a critical detected bacteria in the food industry. Huang et al. [41] found that the TaqMan-MGB probe RT-PCR method established for the *coa* (encoding coagulase) gene of *S. aureus* can enhance the speed and sensitivity of food detection. Multiplex PCR is a PCR reaction that simultaneously amplifies two or more DNA sequences from the same sample [42]. In a study by Schmitz et al. [43] a multiplex PCR on bacteria colonies chosen directly from agar plates without prior DNA preparation is described. In parallel, specific primers were used to detect staphylococcal genes *coa* and *mecA*. Tsai et al. [44] applied multiple PCR technology to detect *Staphylococcus* and *Vibrio vulnificus* in blood and tissue samples of 99 patients with surgically confirmed necrotizing fasciitis (NF) of the extremities. These techniques can be time-consuming and require trained operators who are familiar with the procedure. Therefore, it is interesting to develop a fast, simple, and consistent technology to identify and distinguish between different bacterial species and serotypes.

4.1.2 Isothermal nucleic acid amplification technology

Classical nucleic acid amplification technology has multiple thermal cycling steps, requires strict laboratory conditions, and relies on the use of high-precision instruments that are difficult to miniaturize. The isothermal amplification technology can perform accurate and rapid analysis on site, and is more suitable for integration into miniaturized systems [45]. Loop-mediated isothermal amplification (LAMP) technology was created by Notomi et al. in 2000 [46]. It is a nucleic acid amplification technology that can perform rapid, specific and sensitive detection of target sequences under isothermal conditions. Yin et al. [47] utilize LAMP technology combined with lateral flow assay (LFA) to simultaneously detect *S. aureus sea* and *seb* genes. Strand displacement amplification (SDA) is an enzymatic reaction-based DNA in vitro amplification technology [48]. After the initial thermal denaturation of the dsDNA target, it only needs to reach 37°C for the reaction. Cai et al. [49] reported an SDA-based biosensor for the detection of *S. aureus*. The aptamer was immobilized on streptavidin-modified magnetic beads as a biorecognition molecule, and then bound to its complementary ssDNA. When *S. aureus* is present, the aptamer binds to it, releasing complementary DNA into the solution and detecting pathogenic microorganisms by SDA amplification. The limit of detection (LOD) of the sensor was 8 CFU/ml, and the recovery rate was more than 93.9%. The time-consuming amplification step was optimized from 2 h to 45 min. Although the reaction time was longer compared to other amplification reactions, it had high sensitivity and easy-to-reach reaction temperature advantages. In addition, there are room temperature amplification technologies such as recombinase polymerase amplification (RPA), rolling circle amplification (RCA), simultaneous amplification and testing (SAT), etc.

4.2 Immunoassay

Immunology-based rapid detection technologies for microorganisms include Immune Fluorescence Assay (IFA), Enzyme-linked Immunosorbent Assay (ELISA), Chemiluminescence Immunoassay (CLIA), Radio Immunoassay (RIA), Immunomagnetic Separation (IMS), and Immune Colloidal Gold (ICG) technique, etc. Among them, IMS is a technology that uses the magnetic responsiveness of the magnetic beads to enrich and separate the target substances by coating the recognition substances such as antigens and antibodies on the superparamagnetic nanomagnetic beads with a specific particle size range. The technical operation is simple and fast, with high specificity and sensitivity. Currently, it has been extensively used in protein and nucleic acid purification, cell separation and pathogen detection, such as Multiple Polymerase Chain Reaction (MPCR), Recombinase Polymerase Amplification (RPA), and Loop-Mediated Isothermal Amplification (LAMP). Zhou et al. [50] use avidin-labeled magnetic beads and biotin-labeled SPA monoclonal antibodies to prepare immunomagnetic beads to enrich *S. aureus* from sputum, which is then combined with MPCR to detect the *mecA* gene and *femA* gene of MRSA strains in sputum samples. The detection of MRSA strains has advantages in terms of detection rate, sensitivity and specificity, especially because the detection time can be shortened from 48–72 h to 4–6 h. The most common application of immunoassay techniques is in the detection of *Staphylococcus* toxin. Based on the existing ELISA method, Chang et al. successfully constructed a new staphylococcal enterotoxin A (SEA) detection method for microscale solid phase extraction MSPE-ELISA on magnetic microspheres modified with staphylococcal enterotoxin A (SEA) as an aptamer and introduced solid magnetic phase extraction technology. The sensitivity of magnitude is higher as compared to ELISA kits, enabling the high-sensitivity detection of SEA trace amounts in actual samples. Shan et al. [51] used a carboxyl-modified fluorescent microsphere (PSA-R6G) to immobilize a monoclonal antibody against *S. aureus* as a capture probe. A fluorescein isothiocyanate (FITC)-labeled *S. aureus* secondary fluorescein antibody served as a sensitive reporter antibody. After double labeling with R6G and FITC, multiparameter flow cytometry analysis observed the enriched *S. aureus*. Zhao et al. [52] use vancomycin-immobilized gold nanoparticles (VAN-Au NPs) as the first recognition factor to capture *S. aureus*, and use the second recognition agent of porcine immunoglobulin G (IgG) to ensure its specificity. A novel sandwich-based lateral flow assay (LFA) for highly sensitive and selective detection of *S. aureus*. Tarisse et al. [53] developed an immunoassay that detects the staphylococcal enterotoxins SEA, SEG, SEH, and SEI with high sensitivity and specificity.

4.3 Mass spectrometry

The molecular weight and structure of different biomolecules, such as proteins, nucleic acids, and polysaccharides, can be analyzed using matrix-assisted laser desorption ionization-time of flight mass spectrometry (MALDI-TOF MS) technology. The basic principle behind matrix-assisted laser desorption is as follows: after the matrix and the sample form an eutectic, the matrix and the sample absorb laser energy to desorb the sample, and charge transfer between the matrix and the sample occurs to ionize the sample molecules. The mass-to-charge ratio of ions is proportional, and the mass-to-charge ratio can be measured according to the flight time to the detector, and a characteristic fingerprint can be obtained through software processing [54]. MALDI-TOF MS technology has the characteristics of rapidity, accuracy, sensitivity and automation [55], and gradually occupies an important position in the identification of microbiology laboratories [56]. Rychert et al. [57] conducted a multicenter study on Gram-positive aerobic bacteria, and the results showed that in 1146 Gram-positive bacteria samples, the accuracy rate at the species level was 92.8%, and the accuracy at the genus level could reach 95.5%. The time required for MALDI-TOF MS to obtain identification results has been shortened from 5 to 48 h or even longer via traditional biochemical methods to less than 6 min per sample, and the cost of reagents for single-sample detection has been reduced to less than 1/4 of traditional methods. The overall identification accuracy of MALDI-TOF MS is >90%, which is higher than that of conventional methods (80–85%); in addition, MALDI-TOF MS is easy to operate, which significantly shortens the time for professional and technical training of personnel [58, 59]. MALDI-TOF MS can also be used to analyze the antibiotic resistance of bacteria. The advantages of MALDI-TOF MS are good specificity and short experimental time as compared with conventional antibiotic susceptibility testing (AST) [60, 61]. MOLDI-TOF MS can also quickly differentiate between MRSA and MSSA [62, 63]. The most essential characteristic peaks for distinguishing MRSA and methicillin-sensitive *S. aureus* (MSSA) are at the mass spectrum peaks of 3279, 6485, 6555, and 3299 m/z [64].

4.4 Genome sequencing

In 1977, Sanger et al. [65] invented the dideoxyribonucleotide end termination method, and Maxam and Gilbert [66] developed the chemical degradation method, which marked the birth of the next generation of sequencing technology. Sanger sequencing is the standard technology and its length can be up to 1000 bp and the accuracy is almost 100%, but it has the disadvantages of low throughput, high cost, and long time. Next-generation sequencing (NGS) came into being. Next-generation sequencing platforms mainly include the Roche 454 sequencing platform based on microemulsion PCR and pyrosequencing technology, the Illumina sequencing platform based on bridge PCR and fluorescent reversible terminator sequencing-by-synthesis, the SOLID sequencing platform based on microemulsion PCR and oligonucleotide ligation sequencing, and the Ion Torrent PGM and Proton semiconductor sequencing platforms [67].

In 2014, Wilson et al. [68] reported the world's first case of an infectious disease diagnosed by next-generation sequencing technology. Since then, NGS technology has been gradually recognized and promoted, providing ideas for the diagnosis of unknown pathogens in clinical practice [69] NGS is the most widely used method for high-throughput, massively parallel sequencing of thousands to billions of DNA fragments simultaneously [70]. The third-generation sequencing technology is divided into single-molecule real-time (SMRT) sequencing and nanopore single-molecule sequencing according to different sequencing principles. Gene sequencing can obtain the genomic information of pure colonies and the genomic information of mixed specimens so that highly related lineages can be distinguished with the resolution and precision that other methods lack. Gene sequencing can obtain nearly complete bacterial DNA information, including species, drug-resistance genes, virulence factors, mobile elements, etc. The molecular epidemiology and transmission mechanisms of strains are critical to understanding the occurrence and development of various diseases [71]. The widespread availability of genetic sequencing technology has enabled more detailed studies of MRSA transmission patterns, including analysis of past undocumented transmission and comprehensive, complicated strain evolution [72–74]. In addition, gene sequencing plays a significant role in the study of MRSA colonization and infection [75].

Moore et al. [76] demonstrated that Whole Genome Sequencing (WGS) has a high resolution for strains that other methods cannot distinguish in MRSA colonization and infection studies. WGS is a comprehensive method that analyzes the entire genomic DNA of a cell at once by using sequencing technology. At present, NGS technology still lacks unified laboratory testing operation specifications, and exogenous nucleic acid contamination will likely lead to false positive results, which will seriously affect clinical diagnosis. NGS can detect two or more non-pathogenic bacteria in the same specimen. The analysis may be because NGS has high sensitivity and the nucleic acid residues of non-specimen pathogens with low sequence numbers or dead pathogens are detected together, which is very likely to lead to misjudgment by clinicians, though NGS results lack recognized interpretation. However, the relationship between sequencing results and treatment is unclear, and drug-resistance genes are difficult to detect, so it still needs to be supplemented with drug susceptibility testing. In summary, NGS technology plays an essential role in identifying pathogens and guiding clinical treatment. With the continuous improvement of NGS detection platforms and the proposal of relevant interpretation, NGS technology will be widely used on standards to guide clinical diagnosis and treatment.

5. Raman spectroscopy in *Staphylococcus* identifications

5.1 Principles of Raman scattering effects

Raman scattering is an inelastic scattering phenomenon caused by light striking the surface of a material, revealed by Indian scientist Chandrasekhara Venkata Raman in 1928 [77]. When the molecules of the detected object interact with the incident light photons of the monochromatic beam, elastic and inelastic collisions can occur simultaneously. The scattering mode in which the optical frequency does not change is called Rayleigh scattering. The photon transfers energy to the molecule during an inelastic collision; after it changes direction, some of this energy is transferred to the molecule (Stokes scattering), or the vibration and rotational energy of the molecule is transferred to the photon (Anti-Stokes scattering), changing the frequency of the photon (Raman scattering) [78]. Because Raman scattering can reflect the molecular vibration and vibration-rotation energy level of substances, it is used in molecular structure analysis. However, due to the extremely low scattering efficiency of inelastic scattering, the scattered light intensity is one millionth to one billionth of the incident light intensity, which greatly limits the application of Raman spectroscopy in material analysis and detection, and surface-enhanced Raman spectroscopy was then discovered and developed.

5.2 Surface-enhanced Raman spectroscopy

In 1974, Fleischmann et al. [79] found that the pyridine molecules adsorbed on the rough silver electrode surface had a significant Raman scattering effect. In 1977, after extensive experimental research and theoretical calculation, Jeanmarie et al. [80] named this enhancement effect related to rough metal surfaces such as silver (Ag), gold (Au), and copper (Cu) as the surface-enhanced Raman scattering effect, and the corresponding technology was called surface-enhanced Raman spectroscopy (SERS).

The Raman scattering signal of pyridine molecules adsorbed on the rough metal silver surface is enhanced by about 6 orders of magnitude compared to the Raman scattering signal of pyridine molecules in solution, which provides the possibility for the detection of biological macromolecules. The principle of SERS is explained mainly through two mechanisms: chemical enhancement and electromagnetic enhancement. The chemical mechanism (CM) describes the electronic interaction between substrates and adsorbed molecules and offers a small enhancement magnitude 10^2–10^3. The electromagnetic enhancement (EM) mechanism contributes by increasing the electromagnetic field near plasmonic structures caused by incident light excitation of a localized surface plasmon resonance (LSPR). Plasmonic nanomaterials are those in which incident electromagnetic radiation from light can coherently excite conduction electrons to oscillate collectively at metal/dielectric interfaces. The large SERS enhancement factor (EF) generated from EM contribution to plasmonic nanomaterials is in the magnitude of 10^{10}–10^{14} [81] which is significant for the detection of single molecules [82]. Among them, electromagnetic enhancement receives more attention and acknowledges extensive research work. Label-free SERS detection technology has developed into a research hotspot in the field of microbiology due to its advantages of no need for too much preliminary preparation, non-invasive and short detection time, and excellent application prospects in bacterial detection.

5.3 SERS spectra of staphylococcal bacteria

The complex biological meaning and structural information contained in Raman spectra result from the vibrational and rotational frequencies of molecules in the sample. The vibration frequencies of biomolecules such as nucleic acids, proteins, lipids, and carbohydrates in bacteria are different, and they appear as unique peaks in Raman spectra. "Full biometric fingerprints" can be used as a basis for distinguishing different bacteria. Efrima et al. [83] used SERS for bacterial detection, distinguishing Gram-positive and Gram-negative bacteria through the difference in SERS profiles on the cell membrane surface. Since then, the application of SERS in bacterial detection, identification, and classification has received rapid attention. Rebrošová et al. [84] detected 54 *S. epidermidis* and 51 *Candida parapsilosis* strains from Mueller-Hinton agar plates using Raman spectroscopy with an accuracy of 96.1% and 98.9%, respectively. Tang et al. [85] applied two deep learning methods, Convolutional Neural Networks (CNN) and Long Short-Term Memory (LSTM), for SERS detection of 117 *staphylococcal* strains belonging to 9 species of *Staphylococcus*, with an accuracy of 98.21% and 94.33%, and Area Under Curve (AUC) values of 99.93% and 99.83%, respectively [85]. In addition, *Staphylococcus wornerii*, *S. hominis*, and *Staphylococcus korea* have unique peaks at 1003 cm^{-1}. *Staphylococcus xylinum* and *Staphylococcus squirrels* have special peaks at 1089 and 1093 cm^{-1} [85]. Rebrošová et al. [86] reported that Raman spectroscopy analysis of 277 staphylococcus strains of 16 species, including *S. aureus* and *S. epidermidis*, revealed that the total accuracy of inputting a spectrum was over 99%, and even reached 100% for a few strains, indicating that SERS is a reliable tool for the identification of *Staphylococci*. The most common *S. aureus* Raman peaks are primarily at 731 cm^{-1} [87], which is produced by glycosidic linkages and originates from the abundant peptidoglycan in the cell wall. The other two main Raman peaks at 958 and 1050 cm^{-1} are protein C-O groups. The typical peak of saturated lipids at 1458 cm^{-1} comes from the lipids on the cell wall, while the characteristic peaks of the C-N group are from proteins, peptides, and amino acids on the cell wall [88].

In addition to achieving bacterial classification, SERS technology offers the potential to discriminate various bacterial species that belong to the same family. You et al. [89] used 30 cases of *S. aureus* ATCC25923 and MRSA as the sample training set and 6 cases of ATCC25923 and MRSA as the test set, based on the Principal Component Analysis (PCA) combined linear discriminant analysis (LDA) model for SERS detection. The classification accuracies of ATCC25923 and MRSA on the training and test sets are 76.67% and 75%, respectively according to the PCA-LDA model [89]. In another work, the Ayala team [90] used the SERS technique to differentiate wild-type *S. aureus* and mutant strains lacking carotenoid production. These results confirm the great potential of SERS in identifying *S. aureus*. The feasibility of Raman microscopy has been demonstrated to be able to discriminate various genetically distinct forms of a single bacterial species in situ. The rapid differentiation of resistant and susceptible bacteria can be achieved by collecting the Raman spectral signals of the two and combining them with chemometric methods. In the work of Potluri et al. [91] the PCR and SERS technologies were combined to detect the MRSA-specific genes *mecA* and *femA*, and had good identification of MRSA and MSSA. In identifying MRSA and MSSA, Ciloglu et al. [92] used SERS combined with machine learning techniques for analysis, and the classification accuracy was achieved at 97.8%. In their other work [93], a Sparse Autoencoder (SAE)-based Deep Neural Network (DNN) algorithm was used to analyze and extract features from raw spectral data and classify MRSA and MSSA bacteria with 97.66% accuracy. SERS can be used to analyze the target of drug action and explore the mechanism of antibiotic-resistant, bacteriostatic and bactericidal actions. After the bacteria are treated with drugs, the bacteria are freeze-dried, and the Raman spectrum information of single cells is collected by Raman microscopy. Microscopic imaging can detect the number of drugs entering cells and drug targets, as well as measure the kinetics of drug uptake in cells and point out interactions [94].

5.4 Raman spectroscopy preprocessing

Raman spectral signals inevitably receive external interference during the acquisition process, such as the mechanical vibration of the instrument itself, cosmic noise, and autofluorescence to a certain extent, which prevents the rapid and accurate analysis of spectral data [95]. Therefore, before formal data analysis, the original Raman signal needs to be preprocessed to eliminate unfavorable factors in the analysis process. Preprocessing can be regarded as a key step in spectral data analysis and is mainly divided into spike removal, smoothing denoising, baseline correction, and vector normalization. For peak removal, when collecting Raman spectra, random, narrow and strong spectral signals appear in the spectral fingerprint due to the random appearance of electronic signals from cosmic particles on CCD or complementary metal-oxide-semiconductor detectors. The existence of spikes will mask other useful information to a great extent; therefore, spike removal is necessary. In general, spikes rarely appear at the same shift in the Raman spectrum of the same sample [96]. In this regard, we can judge whether there is a spike by visually inspecting and comparing the difference in abnormal intensity between different spectral curves [97]. In addition, setting the signal intensity threshold and deriving the spectral data can also achieve the purpose of removing spikes [98]. For the electronic noise composed of cosmic noise, flicker noise, and thermal noise, it will randomly appear in multiple positions of the spectral curve in an unpredictable form, which has a large impact on the quality of Raman spectroscopy data. Savitzky–Golay (S-G) filtering is one of the most commonly used preprocessing methods in the process of smoothing and denoising Raman spectra [99, 100].

This method can keep the shape and width of the signal unchanged while filtering the noise, so as to meet the processing requirements of Raman spectral data in different situations [101]. As one of the recognized best processing steps in Raman spectrum analysis preprocessing [96], baseline correction is used to deal with the continuous distortion caused by uncontrollable factors during Raman spectrum acquisition, such as removing substrate-related Raman signals [99] and fluorescence signals generated by the sample itself [102]. Commonly used methods are asymmetric weighted penalized least squares (arPLS) algorithm [103], adaptive iterative weighted penalized least squares (airPLS) algorithm and polynomial fitting [104]. Normalization is the last step of preprocessing [105]. It is used to deal with the situation of large signal strength caused by uneven sample distribution, laser power difference, experimental environment interference and other factors [104]. Vector normalization is one of the most commonly used normalization methods in Raman spectral analysis [97, 106], It is used to control the difference in Raman signal intensity levels by mapping the data to a range of 0 to 1 for processing [107]. It is worth noting that the order of preprocessing is not fixed and each step does not necessarily need to be performed. When applying to our own experimental data, we need to observe the interaction between each step of preprocessing, and choose the best combination of preprocessing according to the feedback between different preprocessing methods.

5.5 Machine learning analysis of SERS spectra

Data learning aims to convert Raman spectral signals into computer-recognizable abstract feature information. For previously preprocessed spectral data, we need to use more advanced methods based on machine learning algorithms. Machine Learning (ML) is a method of observing existing data, extracting the rules, and then applying them to unknown samples [98]. Traditional Raman spectrum classification and recognition usually use machine-learning algorithms to model and analyze, but the analysis process of this method is relatively complicated, and it needs to go through operations such as preprocessing and feature extraction. In recent years, deep learning has become a hot research topic. Deep learning is to learn features from large-scale raw datasets and to build predictive models directly. There are many deep learning algorithms, including convolutional neural networks (CNN), fully connected networks, and residual neural networks (ResNet), etc. It has decent performance in mining local features of data and extracting international training highlights [108], and its ability to classify and identify data far exceeds that of traditional multivariate statistical analysis algorithms. Wang et al. [109] prepared positively charged nano-silver-based SERS samples combined with the CNN algorithm for rapid identification of drug resistance in *S. aureus*. Several classifications have achieved good results for the high-intensity SERS fingerprints collected in 107 cells/ml bacterial solution, among which shallow CNN, ResNet25, SVM and Logistic regression all achieved 100% classification accuracy [109]. When the traditional machine learning algorithms SVM, Logistic regression, RF and KNN were used to analyze low-intensity SERS fingerprints collected from low-concentration bacterial solutions of 105 cells/ml and 102 cells/ml, the average recognition accuracy dropped below 80% [109] whereas the shallow layer created by the study CNN achieves 94.5% recognition accuracy, which is more than 25% higher than other ordinary methods [109]. In addition, the SERS combined CNN detection method also achieved good results in identifying MRSA and MSSA. Ho et al. [110] apply deep learning methods to identify 30 common bacterial pathogens. The average separation level was more than 82% accurate at low SNR spectra, and an antibiotic treatment identification accuracy of 97.0 ± 0.3% was achieved [110]. The deep learning method distinguishes between MRSA and MSSA isolates with an accuracy of 89 ± 0.1% [110]. Additionally, Tang et al. studied 9 different *Staphylococci*, and constructed 8 different machine learning algorithms and 2 deep learning algorithms for the classification and prediction of all the staphylococcal strains [94]. By calculating and comparing the evaluation indicators of different models, it is found that the deep learning algorithm CNN has the best performance (ACC = 98.21%), and the AUC is also the largest (99.93%) [94]. The results show that the deep learning algorithm has strong classification and prediction capabilities in the detection of bacterial pathogens through surface enhanced Raman spectroscopy.

6. Conclusion and perspectives

With the continuous development of science and technology, the detection methods of *Staphylococcus* have become more and more diverse, but they all have their advantages and disadvantages. Although the traditional cultivation method is the gold standard, the cultivation time is long, the steps are cumbersome and the technical requirements of the testing personnel are high. Molecular-level identification methods such as PCR, mass spectrometry, and whole-genome sequencing have high sensitivity and specificity with short turn-around time, and can directly detect clinical samples but these techniques have steep learning curves and are expensive. In order to better make up for the shortcomings of various methods, this paper introduces surface-enhanced Raman technology, which has the advantages of low cost, simple operation, label-free, non-invasiveness, high sensitivity, and high specificity in bacterial identification and drug resistance detection, which has great application potential in the near future.

Glossary	Abbreviations
MRSA	methicillin-resistant *Staphylococcus aureus*
SERS	surface enhanced Raman spectroscopy
CPS	coagulase positive Staphylococcus
CNS	coagulase-negative Staphylococcus
SCVs	Small colony variants
MSM	mannitol salt medium
SPA	Staphylococcus Protein A
SSSS	staphylococcal scalded skin syndrome
TSS	toxic shock syndrome
SFP	*S. aureus* food poisoning
SEs	staphylococcal enterotoxins
CLSI	Clinical and Laboratory Standards Institute
EUCAST	European Committee for Antimicrobial Susceptibility Testing
K-B	Kirby-Bauer
MIC	minimum inhibitory concentration

Glossary	Abbreviations
MHB	Mueller Hinton Broth
MBC	minimal bactericidal concentration
VISA	vancomycin-intermediate *S. aureus*
VRSA	vancomycin-resistant *S. aureus*
PCR	Polymerase chain reaction
NF	necrotizing fasciitis
LAMP	Loop-mediated isothermal amplification
LFA	lateral flow assay
SDA	Strand displacement amplification
RPA	recombinase polymerase amplification
RCA	rolling circle amplification
SAT	simultaneous amplification and testing
IFA	immune fluorescence assay
ELISA	enzyme-linked immunosorbent assay
CLIA	chemiluminescence immunoassay
RIA	radioimmunoassay
IMS	immunomagnetic separation
ICG	immune colloidal gold
SEA	staphylococcal enterotoxin A
MSPE	microscale solid phase extraction
FITC	fluorescein isothiocyanate
MALDI-TOF MS	matrix-assisted laser desorption ionization-time of flight mass spectrometry
AST	antibiotic susceptibility testing
MSSA	methicillin-sensitive *Staphylococcus aureus*
NGS	next-generation sequencing
SMRT	single-molecule real-time
CM	chemical mechanism
EM	electromagnetic enhancement
LSPR	localized surface plasmon resonance
EF	enhancement factor
CNN	convolutional neural networks
LSTM	long short-term memory
AUC	area under curve
PCA	principal component analysis
LDA	linear discriminant analysis
SAE	sparse autoencoder
DNN	deep neural network

Author details

Xue-Di Zhang[1,2] †, Bin Gu[3] †, Muhammad Usman[3] †, Jia-Wei Tang[3], Zheng-Kang Li[4], Xin-Qiang Zhang[4], Jia-Wei Yan[2*] and Liang Wang[4*]

1 Laboratory Medicine, Medical Technology School of Xuzhou Medical University, Xuzhou, Jiangsu Province, China

2 Laboratory Medicine, Xuzhou Infectious Diseases Hospital, Xuzhou, Jiangsu Province, China

3 Department of Intelligent Medical Engineering, School of Medical Informatics and Engineering, Xuzhou Medical University, Xuzhou, Jiangsu Province, China

4 Laboratory Medicine, Guangdong Provincial People's Hospital, Guangdong Academy of Medical Sciences, Guangzhou, Guangdong Province, China

*Address all correspondence to: jiawei.yanh@foxmail.com
and healthscienc@foxmail.com

† These authors contributed equally to the study.

References

[1] Schlecht LM, Peters BM, Krom BP, Freiberg JA, Hänsch GM, Filler SG, et al. Systemic *Staphylococcus aureus* infection mediated by Candida albicans hyphal invasion of mucosal tissue. Microbiology (Reading). 2015;**161**(Pt 1):168-181

[2] Parte AC, Sardà Carbasse J, Meier-Kolthoff JP, Reimer LC, Göker M. List of prokaryotic names with standing in nomenclature (LPSN) moves to the DSMZ. International Journal of Systematic and Evolutionary Microbiology. 2020;**70**(11):5607-5612

[3] Schmidt TM. Encyclopedia of Microbiology. USA, Cambridge, Massachusetts: Academic Press; 2009

[4] Del Giudice P. Skin infections caused by *Staphylococcus aureus*. Acta Dermato-Venereologica. 2020;**100**(9):adv00110

[5] Lina G, Piémont Y, Godail-Gamot F, Bes M, Peter MO, Gauduchon V, et al. Involvement of Panton-valentine leukocidin-producing *Staphylococcus aureus* in primary skin infections and pneumonia. Clinical Infectious Diseases. 1999;**29**(5):1128-1132

[6] Otto M. *Staphylococcus epidermidis*—The 'accidental' pathogen. Nature Reviews. Microbiology. 2009;**7**(8):555-567

[7] Argudín M, Mendoza MC, Rodicio MR. Food poisoning and *Staphylococcus aureus* enterotoxins. Toxins (Basel). 2010;**2**(7):1751-1773

[8] Tuffs SW, Goncheva MI, Xu SX, Craig HC, Kasper KJ, Choi J, et al. Superantigens promote *Staphylococcus aureus* bloodstream infection by eliciting pathogenic interferon-gamma production. Proceedings of the National Academy of Sciences of the United States of America. 2022;**119**(8):e2115987119

[9] Hovelius B, Mårdh PA. *Staphylococcus saprophyticus* as a common cause of urinary tract infections. Reviews of Infectious Diseases. 1984;**6**(3):328-337

[10] Hamdan-Partida A, Sainz-Espuñes T, Bustos-Martínez J. Characterization and persistence of *Staphylococcus aureus* strains isolated from the anterior nares and throats of healthy carriers in a Mexican community. Journal of Clinical Microbiology. 2010;**48**(5):1701-1705

[11] Hamdan-Partida A, González-García S, de la Rosa GE, Bustos-Martínez J. Community-acquired methicillin-resistant *Staphylococcus aureus* can persist in the throat. International Journal of Medical Microbiology. 2018;**308**(4):469-475

[12] González-García S, Hamdan-Partida A, Bustos-Hamdan A, Bustos-Martínez J. Factors of nasopharynx that favor the colonization and persistence of *staphylococcus aureus*. In: Zhou X, Zhang Z, editors. Pharynx-Diagnosis and Treatment. London: IntechOpen; 2021. pp. 75-81

[13] Boucher HW, Corey GR. Epidemiology of methicillin-resistant *Staphylococcus aureus*. Clinical Infectious Diseases. 2008;**46**(Suppl 5):S344-S349

[14] F G. The genera Staphylococcus and Macrococcus. The Prokaryotes. 2006;**2006**:5-75

[15] Visansirikul S, Kolodziej SA, Demchenko AV. *Staphylococcus aureus* capsular polysaccharides: A structural

and synthetic perspective. Organic & Biomolecular Chemistry. 2020;**18**(5): 783-798

[16] Bautista-Trujillo GU, Solorio-Rivera JL, Rentería-Solórzano I, Carranza-GermánSI,Bustos-MartínezJA, Arteaga-Garibay RI, et al. Performance of culture media for the isolation and identification of *Staphylococcus aureus* from bovine mastitis. Journal of Medical Microbiology. 2013;**62**(Pt 3):369-376

[17] Melter O, Radojevič B. Small colony variants of *Staphylococcus aureus*—Review. Folia Microbiologia (Praha). 2010;**55**(6):548-558

[18] Moraveji Z, Tabatabaei M, Shirzad Aski H, Khoshbakht R. Characterization of hemolysins of Staphylococcus strains isolated from human and bovine, southern Iran. Iranian Journal of Veterinary Research. 2014;**15**(4):326-330

[19] Chen HZ, Lin GW. Shiyong Neikexue. Beijing: Beijing People's Medical Publishing House; 2009

[20] Kourtis AP, Hatfield K, Baggs J, Mu Y, See I, Epson E, et al. Vital signs: Epidemiology and recent trends in methicillin-resistant and in methicillin-susceptible *Staphylococcus aureus* bloodstream infections—United States. Morbidity and Mortality Weekly Report. 2019;**68**(9):214-219

[21] Kloos WE, Musselwhite MS. Distribution and persistence of Staphylococcus and Micrococcus species and other aerobic bacteria on human skin. Applied Microbiology. 1975;**30**(3):381-385

[22] Rupp ME, Soper DE, Archer GL. Colonization of the female genital tract with *Staphylococcus saprophyticus*. Journal of Clinical Microbiology. 1992;**30**(11):2975-2979

[23] Bush LM. Best alternative to vancomycin for serious methicillin-resistant *Staphylococcus aureus* infections: let's just say it. Clinical Infectious Diseases. 2011;**53**(9):965-966

[24] Leonard FC, Markey BK. Meticillin-resistant *Staphylococcus aureus* in animals: A review. Veterinary Journal. 2008;**175**(1):27-36

[25] Ghahramani G. Superficial Staphylococcal and Streptococcal Infections. InInpatient Dermatology. Cham: Springer; 2018

[26] Morelli P, De Alessandri A, Manno G, Marchese A, Bassi M, Lobello R, et al. Characterization of *Staphylococcus aureus* small colony variant strains isolated from Italian patients attending a regional cystic fibrosis care Centre. The New Microbiologica. 2015;**38**(2):235-243

[27] Proctor RA, Kriegeskorte A, Kahl BC, Becker K, Löffler B, Peters G. *Staphylococcus aureus* small Colony variants (SCVs): A road map for the metabolic pathways involved in persistent infections. Frontiers in Cellular and Infection Microbiology. 2014;**4**:99

[28] Bui LMG, Turnidge JD, Kidd SP. The induction of *Staphylococcus aureus* biofilm formation or small Colony variants is a strain-specific response to host-generated chemical stresses. Microbes and Infection. 2015;**17**(1):77-82

[29] Levy J, Van Laethem Y, Verhaegen G, Perpête C, Butzler JP, Wenzel RP. Contaminated enteral nutrition solutions as a cause of nosocomial bloodstream infection: A study using plasmid fingerprinting. Journal of Parenteral and Enteral Nutrition. 1989;**13**(3):228-234

[30] Fan Y, Wang X, Li L, Yao Z, Chen S, Ye X. Potential relationship between phenotypic and molecular characteristics in revealing livestock-associated *Staphylococcus aureus* in Chinese humans without occupational livestock contact. Frontiers in Microbiology. 2016;**7**:1517

[31] Turner NA, Sharma-Kuinkel BK, Maskarinec SA, Eichenberger EM, Shah PP, Carugati M, et al. Methicillin-resistant *Staphylococcus aureus*: An overview of basic and clinical research. Nature Reviews. Microbiology. 2019;**17**(4):203-218

[32] Hiramatsu K, Ito T, Tsubakishita S, Sasaki T, Takeuchi F, Morimoto Y, et al. Genomic basis for methicillin resistance in *Staphylococcus aureus*. Infection & Chemotherapy. 2013;**45**(2):117-136

[33] Ballhausen B, Kriegeskorte A, Schleimer N, Peters G, Becker K. The mecA homolog mecC confers resistance against β-lactams in *Staphylococcus aureus* irrespective of the genetic strain background. Antimicrobial Agents and Chemotherapy. 2014;**58**(7):3791-3798

[34] Kim C, Milheiriço C, Gardete S, Holmes MA, Holden MT, de Lencastre H, et al. Properties of a novel PBP2A protein homolog from *Staphylococcus aureus* strain LGA251 and its contribution to the β-lactam-resistant phenotype. The Journal of Biological Chemistry. 2012;**287**(44):36854-36863

[35] Peacock SJ, Paterson GK. Mechanisms of methicillin resistance in *Staphylococcus aureus*. Annual Review of Biochemistry. 2015;**84**:577-601

[36] Li X, Xiong Y, Fan X, Feng P, Tang H, Zhou T. The role of femA regulating gene on methicillin-resistant *Staphylococcus aureus* clinical isolates. Médecine et Maladies Infectieuses. 2012;**42**(5):218-225

[37] Berger-Bächi B, Rohrer S. Factors influencing methicillin resistance in staphylococci. Archives of Microbiology. 2002;**178**(3):165-171

[38] Wayne PA. Performance Standards for Antimicrobial Susceptibility Testing, 32nd Informational Supplement. M100-S32. Malvern, PA: Clinical and Laboratory Standards Institute; 2022

[39] Okolie CE. Real-time PCR to identify staphylococci and assay for virulence from blood. Methods in Molecular Biology. 2017;**1616**:183-207

[40] Yang XY, Liu R, Mu XY, Yang XY, Liu R, Mu XY. Shishi yingguang dingliang PCR fa jianding jianding nai jiayang xilin jinhuang se putao qiujun xiaoguo guancha. Shandong Medical Journal. 2016;**6**:80-81

[41] Huang FG, Yue YH, Huang JC, Zhang XL. Jinhuang se putao qiujun coa jiyin shishi yingguang PCR de jianli ji yingyong yanjiu. Chinese Journal of Health Laboratory Technology. 2017;**27**(94-6):100

[42] Korbie D, Trau M. Multiplex PCR design for scalable resequencing. Methods in Molecular Biology. 2022;**2392**:143-158

[43] Schmitz FJ, Mackenzie CR, Hofmann B, Verhoef J, Finken-Eigen M, Heinz HP, et al. Specific information concerning taxonomy, pathogenicity and methicillin resistance of staphylococci obtained by a multiplex PCR. Journal of Medical Microbiology. 1997;**46**(9):773-778

[44] Tsai YH, Chen PH, Yu PA, Chen CL, Kuo LT, Huang KC. A multiplex PCR assay for detection of *Vibrio vulnificus*, *Aeromonas hydrophila*, methicillin-resistant *Staphylococcus aureus*, *Streptococcus pyogenes*, and *Streptococcus*

agalactiae from the isolates of patients with necrotizing fasciitis. International Journal of Infectious Diseases. 2019;**81**:73-80

[45] Toldrà A, O'Sullivan CK, Campàs M. Detecting harmful algal blooms with isothermal molecular strategies. Trends in Biotechnology. 2019;**37**(12):1278-1281

[46] Notomi T, Okayama H, Masubuchi H, Yonekawa T, Watanabe K, Amino N, et al. Loop-mediated isothermal amplification of DNA. Nucleic Acids Research. 2000;**28**(12):E63

[47] Yin HY, Fang TJ, Wen HW. Combined multiplex loop-mediated isothermal amplification with lateral flow assay to detect sea and seb genes of enterotoxic *Staphylococcus aureus*. Letters in Applied Microbiology. 2016;**63**(1):16-24

[48] Reid MS, Le XC, Zhang H. Exponential isothermal amplification of nucleic acids and assays for proteins, cells, small molecules, and enzyme activities: An EXPAR example. Angewandte Chemie (International Ed. in English). 2018;**57**(37):11856-11866

[49] Cai R, Zhang Z, Chen H, Tian Y, Zhou N. A versatile signal-on electrochemical biosensor for *Staphylococcus aureus* based on triple-helix molecular switch. Sensors and Actuators B: Chemical. 2021;**326**:128842

[50] Zhou LZ, Geng XL, Zhao Q. Tanye nai jiayang xilin jinhuang se putao qiujun kuaisu jiance jiqi linchuang yingyong. Journal of Nantong University Medical Edition. 2017;**37**:322-324

[51] Shan Y, Xu C, Wang M, Zhu Z, Wu FG, Shi Z, et al. Bilinear *Staphylococcus aureus* detection based on suspension immunoassay. Talanta. 2019;**192**:154-159

[52] Zhao M, Yao X, Liu S, Zhang H, Wang L, Yin X, et al. Antibiotic and mammal IgG based lateral flow assay for simple and sensitive detection of *Staphylococcus aureus*. Food Chemistry. 2021;**339**:127955

[53] Tarisse CF, Goulard-Huet C, Nia Y, Devilliers K, Marcé D, Dambrune C, et al. Highly sensitive and specific detection of Staphylococcal enterotoxins SEA, SEG, SEH, and SEI by immunoassay. Toxins (Basel). 2021;**13**(2):130

[54] Croxatto A, Prod'hom G, Greub G. Applications of MALDI-TOF mass spectrometry in clinical diagnostic microbiology. FEMS Microbiology Reviews. 2012;**36**(2):380-407

[55] Doern CD. Integration of technology into clinical practice. Clinics in Laboratory Medicine. 2013;**33**(3):705-729

[56] Biswas S, Rolain JM. Use of MALDI-TOF mass spectrometry for identification of bacteria that are difficult to culture. Journal of Microbiological Methods. 2013;**92**(1):14-24

[57] Rychert J, Burnham CA, Bythrow M, Garner OB, Ginocchio CC, Jennemann R, et al. Multicenter evaluation of the Vitek MS matrix-assisted laser desorption ionization-time of flight mass spectrometry system for identification of gram-positive aerobic bacteria. Journal of Clinical Microbiology. 2013;**51**(7):2225-2231

[58] Bizzini A, Greub G. Matrix-assisted laser desorption ionization time-of-flight mass spectrometry, a revolution in clinical microbial identification. Clinical Microbiology and Infection. 2010;**16**(11):1614-1619

[59] Zhongguo L, Wei S, Zhipu Y, Zhuanjia G. Chinese clinical microbial mass spectrometry consensus

expert group, Chinese Journal of Nosocomiology. 2016;**26**(3):411-419

[60] van Belkum A, Welker M, Pincus D, Charrier JP, Girard V. Matrix-assisted laser desorption ionization time-of-flight mass spectrometry in clinical microbiology: What are the current issues? Annals of Laboratory Medicine. 2017;**37**(6):475-483

[61] Vrioni G, Tsiamis C, Oikonomidis G, Theodoridou K, Kapsimali V, Tsakris A. MALDI-TOF mass spectrometry technology for detecting biomarkers of antimicrobial resistance: Current achievements and future perspectives. Annals of Translational Medicine. 2018;**6**(12):240

[62] Wang YR, Chen Q, Cui SH, Li FQ. Characterization of *Staphylococcus aureus* isolated from clinical specimens by matrix assisted laser desorption/ionization time-of-flight mass spectrometry. Biomedical and Environmental Sciences. 2013;**26**(6):430-436

[63] Hu Y, Cai J, Zhou H. Rapid identification of methicillin-resistant *Staphylococcus aureus* and methicillin-sensitive *Staphylococcus aureus* strains by matrix-assisted laser desorption/ionization time-of-flight mass spectrometry Chinese. Journal of Microbiology and Immunology. 2015;**35**(1):42-45

[64] Wolters M, Rohde H, Maier T, Belmar-Campos C, Franke G, Scherpe S, et al. MALDI-TOF MS fingerprinting allows for discrimination of major methicillin-resistant *Staphylococcus aureus* lineages. International Journal of Medical Microbiology. 2011;**301**(1):64-68

[65] Sanger F, Air GM, Barrell BG, Brown NL, Coulson AR, Fiddes CA, et al. Nucleotide sequence of bacteriophage phi X174 DNA. Nature. 1977;**265**(5596):687-695

[66] Maxam AM, Gilbert W. A new method for sequencing DNA. Proceedings of the National Academy of Sciences of the United States of America. 1977;**74**(2):560-564

[67] Zhang XZ. Xia yidai jiyin cexu jishu xin jinzhan. Journal of Lanzhou University Medical Edition. 2016;**42**:73-80

[68] Wilson MR, Naccache SN, Samayoa E, Biagtan M, Bashir H, Yu G, et al. Actionable diagnosis of neuroleptospirosis by next-generation sequencing. The New England Journal of Medicine. 2014;**370**(25):2408-2417

[69] Reuter JA, Spacek DV, Snyder MP. High-throughput sequencing technologies. Molecular Cell. 2015;**58**(4):586-597

[70] Gu W, Miller S, Chiu CY. Clinical metagenomic next-generation sequencing for pathogen detection. Annual Review of Pathology. 2019;**14**:319-338

[71] Tenover FC, Tickler IA, Le VM, Dewell S, Mendes RE, Goering RV. Updating molecular diagnostics for detecting methicillin-susceptible and methicillin-resistant *Staphylococcus aureus* isolates in blood culture bottles. Journal of Clinical Microbiology. 2019;**57**(11)

[72] Croucher NJ, Didelot X. The application of genomics to tracing bacterial pathogen transmission. Current Opinion in Microbiology. 2015;**23**:62-67

[73] Anjum MF, Marco-Jimenez F, Duncan D, Marín C, Smith RP, Evans SJ. Livestock-associated methicillin-resistant *Staphylococcus aureus* from animals and

animal products in the UK. Frontiers in Microbiology. 2019;**10**:2136

[74] Durand G, Javerliat F, Bes M, Veyrieras JB, Guigon G, Mugnier N, et al. Routine whole-genome sequencing for outbreak investigations of *Staphylococcus aureus* in a National Reference Center. Frontiers in Microbiology. 2018;**9**:511

[75] Senn L, Clerc O, Zanetti G, Basset P, Prod'hom G, Gordon NC, et al. The stealthy superbug: the role of asymptomatic enteric carriage in maintaining a long-term hospital outbreak of ST228 methicillin-resistant *Staphylococcus aureus*. mBio. 2016;7(1):e02039-e02015

[76] Moore G, Cookson B, Gordon NC, Jackson R, Kearns A, Singleton J, et al. Whole-genome sequencing in hierarchy with pulsed-field gel electrophoresis: The utility of this approach to establish possible sources of MRSA cross-transmission. The Journal of Hospital Infection. 2015;**90**(1):38-45

[77] Raman CV. A change of wave-length in light scattering. Nature. 1928;**121**(3051):619

[78] Kneipp K, Kneipp H, Corio P, Brown SD, Shafer K, Motz J, et al. Surface-enhanced and normal stokes and anti-stokes Raman spectroscopy of single-walled carbon nanotubes. Physical Review Letters. 2000;**84**(15):3470-3473

[79] Fleischmann M, Hendra PJ, McQuillan AJ. Raman spectra of pyridine adsorbed at a silver electrode. Chemical Physics Letters. 1974;**26**(2):163-166

[80] Jeanmaire DL, Van Duyne RP. Surface raman spectroelectrochemistry: Part I. Heterocyclic, aromatic, and aliphatic amines adsorbed on the anodized silver slectrode. Journal of Electroanalytical Chemistry and Interfacial Electrochemistry. 1997;**84**(1):1-20

[81] Shan B. Novel SERS labels: Rational design, functional integration and biomedical applications. Coordination Chemistry Reviews. 2018;**371**:11-37

[82] Le Ru EC, Blackie E, Meyer M, Etchegoin PG. Surface enhanced Raman scattering enhancement factors: A comprehensive study. The Journal of Physical Chemistry, C Nanomaterials and Interfaces. 2007;**111**:13794-13803

[83] Zeiri L, Bronk BV, Shabtai Y, Eichler J, Efrima S. Surface-enhanced Raman spectroscopy as a tool for probing specific biochemical components in bacteria. Applied Spectroscopy. 2004;**58**(1):33-40

[84] Rebrošová K, Šiler M, Samek O, Růžička F, Bernatová S, Ježek J, et al. Identification of ability to form biofilm in Candida parapsilosis and *Staphylococcus epidermidis* by Raman spectroscopy. Future Microbiology. 2019;**14**:509-517

[85] Tang JW, Liu QH, Yin XC, Pan YC, Wen PB, Liu X, et al. Comparative analysis of machine learning algorithms on surface enhanced Raman spectra of clinical Staphylococcus species. Frontiers in Microbiology. 2021;**12**:696921

[86] Rebrošová K, Šiler M, Samek O, Růžička F, Bernatová S, Holá V, et al. Rapid identification of staphylococci by Raman spectroscopy. Scientific Reports. 2017;7(1):14846

[87] Chen J, Park B, Eady M. Simultaneous detection and serotyping of salmonellae by immunomagnetic separation and label-free surface-enhanced Raman spectroscopy. Food Analytical Methods. 2017;**10**(9): 3181-3193

[88] Liu Y, Zhou H, Hu Z, Yu G, Yang D, Zhao J. Label and label-free based surface-enhanced Raman scattering for pathogen bacteria detection: A review. Biosensors & Bioelectronics. 2017;**94**:131-140

[89] You HJ, Lu ZH, Shi P. Nami yin rongye jiao jiedao de biaomian zengqiang laman yongyu xijun de jianding yanjiu. Journal of Microbiology. 2019;**39**:76-82

[90] Ayala OD, Wakeman CA, Pence IJ, Gaddy JA, Slaughter JC, Skaar EP, et al. Drug-resistant *Staphylococcus aureus* strains reveal distinct biochemical features with Raman microspectroscopy. ACS Infectious Diseases. 2018;**4**(8):1197-1210

[91] Potluri PR, Rajendran VK, Sunna A, Wang Y. Rapid and specific duplex detection of methicillin-resistant *Staphylococcus aureus* genes by surface-enhanced Raman spectroscopy. Analyst. 2020;**145**(7):2789-2794

[92] Uysal Ciloglu F, Saridag AM, Kilic IH, Tokmakci M, Kahraman M, Aydin O. Identification of methicillin-resistant *Staphylococcus aureus* bacteria using surface-enhanced Raman spectroscopy and machine learning techniques. Analyst. 2020;**145**(23):7559-7570

[93] Ciloglu FU, Caliskan A, Saridag AM, Kilic IH, Tokmakci M, Kahraman M, et al. Drug-resistant *Staphylococcus aureus* bacteria detection by combining surface-enhanced Raman spectroscopy (SERS) and deep learning techniques. Scientific Reports. 2021;**11**(1):18444

[94] Carey PR, Heidari-Torkabadi H. New techniques in antibiotic discovery and resistance: Raman spectroscopy. Annals of the New York Academy of Sciences. 2015;**1354**:67-81

[95] Spectral analysis: A rapid tool for species detection in meat products. Trends in Food Science and Technology. 2017;**62**:59-67

[96] Guo S, Popp J, Bocklitz T. Chemometric analysis in Raman spectroscopy from experimental design to machine learning-based modeling. Nature Protocols. 2021;**16**(12):5426-5459

[97] Yamamoto T, Taylor JN, Koseki S, Koyama K. Classification of food spoilage bacterial species and their sodium chloride, sodium acetate and glycine tolerance using chemometrics analysis and Raman spectroscopy. Journal of Microbiological Methods. 2021;**190**:106326

[98] Makridakis S, Spiliotis E, Assimakopoulos V. Statistical and machine learning forecasting methods: Concerns and ways forward. PLoS One. 2018;**13**(3):e0194889

[99] Bashir S, Nawaz H, Irfan Majeed M, Mohsin M, Nawaz A, Rashid N, et al. Surface-enhanced Raman spectroscopy for the identification of tigecycline-resistant E. coli strains. Spectrochimica Acta. Part A, Molecular and Biomolecular Spectroscopy. 2021;**258**:119831

[100] Naseer K, Saleem M, Ali S, Mirza B, Qazi J. Identification of new spectral signatures from hepatitis C virus infected human sera. Spectrochimica Acta. Part A, Molecular and Biomolecular Spectroscopy. 2019;**222**:117181

[101] Bashir S, Nawaz H, Majeed MI, Mohsin M, Abdullah S, Ali S, et al. Rapid and sensitive discrimination among carbapenem resistant and susceptible E. coli strains using surface enhanced Raman spectroscopy combined with chemometric tools. Photodiagnosis and Photodynamic Therapy. 2021;**34**:102280

[102] Wichmann C, Chhallani M, Bocklitz T, Rösch P, Popp J. Simulation of transportation and storage and

their influence on Raman spectra of bacteria. Analytical Chemistry. 2019;**91**(21):13688-13694

[103] Baek SJ, Park A, Ahn YJ, Choo J. Baseline correction using asymmetrically reweighted penalized least squares smoothing. Analyst. 2015;**140**(1):250-257

[104] Liu Y, Xu J, Tao Y, Fang T, Du W, Ye A. Rapid and accurate identification of marine microbes with single-cell Raman spectroscopy. Analyst. 2020;**145**(9):3297-3305

[105] Kothari R, Fong Y, Storrie-Lombardi MC. Review of laser Raman spectroscopy for surgical breast cancer detection: Stochastic backpropagation neural networks. Sensors (Basel). 2020;**20**(21):6260

[106] Dastgir G, Majeed MI, Nawaz H, Rashid N, Raza A, Ali MZ, et al. Surface-enhanced Raman spectroscopy of polymerase chain reaction (PCR) products of Rifampin resistant and susceptible tuberculosis patients. Photodiagnosis and Photodynamic Therapy. 2022;**38**:102758

[107] Ullah R, Khan S, Chaudhary II, Shahzad S, Ali H, Bilal M. Cost effective and efficient screening of tuberculosis disease with Raman spectroscopy and machine learning algorithms. Photodiagnosis and Photodynamic Therapy. 2020;**32**:101963

[108] Eraslan G, Avsec Ž, Gagneur J, Theis FJ. Deep learning: New computational modelling techniques for genomics. Nature Reviews. Genetics. 2019;**20**(7):389-403

[109] Wang S, Wang CW, Gu B. Biaomian zengqiang laman sanshe jiehe juanji shenjing wangluo yongyu nai jiayang xilin jinhuangse putao qiujun de jingzhun jiance. Linchuang Jianyan Zazhi. 2022;**40**:81-86

[110] Ho CS, Jean N, Hogan CA, Blackmon L, Jeffrey SS, Holodniy M, et al. Rapid identification of pathogenic bacteria using Raman spectroscopy and deep learning. Nature Communications. 2019;**10**(1):4927

Chapter 6

Occurrence of Mastitis in Dairy Herds and the Detection of Virulence Factors in Staphylococci

František Zigo, Zuzana Farkašová, Ibrahim Farag Mohammed Rehan and Ahmed Sayed-Ahmed

Abstract

Mastitis is still a major challenge that affects milk quality. The study is aimed to examine the health of the mammary gland and identify the udder pathogens and virulence factors that caused mastitis in 960 dairy cows and 940 ewes, respectively. We found that Staphylococci and streptococci are the most common causes of mastitis in those dairy animals. Coagulase-negative staphylococci (CoNS), along with the main udder pathogens such as *S. aureus, S. uberis, and S. agalactiae*, are a major concern for dairy animals. The majority of the virulence factors (production of hemolysis, gelatinase, biofilm, ability to hydrolyze DNA, and antibiotic resistance) were found in *S. chromogens, S. warneri, and S. xylosus* isolates from clinical and chronic cases of mastitis. S. aureus and CoNS strains tested by disk diffusion showed 77.0 and 44.2% resistance to one or more antimicrobial classes in mastitic milk samples from dairy cows and ewes, respectively. The presence of a methicillin-resistant gene *mecA* poses serious complications for treatment and indicates a health risk to milk consumers due to the resistance to β-lactam-antibiotics in two isolates of *S. aureus* and two species of CoNS isolated from cows' mastitic milk samples.

Keywords: dairy cows, ewes, mastitis, coagulase-negative staphylococci, biofilm, antibiotics, methicillin resistance gene

1. Introduction

Milk and milk products are important global dietary products, consumed by more than 6 billion people worldwide. In 2019, the recorded milk consumption was 852 million tons, distinguishing the dairy industry as a very profitable market. The milk obtained is a traditional raw material for the production of a range of dairy products, which are unique in their composition, but EU rules emphasize that such products must come from healthy animals, which significantly limits their production and quality [1].

Despite the increasing level of zoohygienic provision of dairy farming, inflammation of the mammary gland-mastitis is still one of the main health problems.

This disease is associated with pain and adversely affects animal health, welfare, milk quality, and the economics of milk production. Direct and indirect losses, caused by mastitis lead to economic losses. For direct losses, we can include treatment costs, discarded milk, labor time, fatalities, and the associated costs with repeated cases of mastitis. Regarding indirect losses, we can include increased culling, decreased milk production, decreased milk quality, loss of premiums, preterm drying-off, animal welfare aspects, and other associated health problems [2, 3]. According to a study by Hogeveen et al. [4], the losses for the global dairy industry are estimated at 16–26 billion euros per year, based on a global population of 271 million dairy cows, with a cost of €61–97 per animal for farmers. In the United States, economically bovine mastitis costs around $2 billion every year. It has also been identified as one of the most economically relevant diseases in Ireland by Animal Health Ireland [5]. In the Netherlands, van Soest et al. [6] estimated the total cost of mastitis in 108 dairy farms, and found that the average total cost of mastitis is €240/lactating cow per year. In addition, failure costs contributed €120/lactating cow per year and preventive costs also contributed another €120/lactating cow per year.

Due to their polyethological origin, infections of the mammary gland are most often caused by a complex of interactions among the host, environment, and infectious agents that result in bovine mastitis, one of the most frequent diseases of dairy cows and ewes (**Figure 1**). Mastitis has a significant impact on global dairy production, reducing both the quality and quantity of milk produced. In comparison with most other animal diseases, mastitis differs by the fact that several diverse kinds of bacteria can cause the infection. These pathogens are capable of invading the udder, multiplying there, and producing harmful, inflammation-causing compounds [7].

Up to this date, more than 137 different organisms have been recognized as causative agents of ruminant intramammary infection (IMI). They include bacteria,

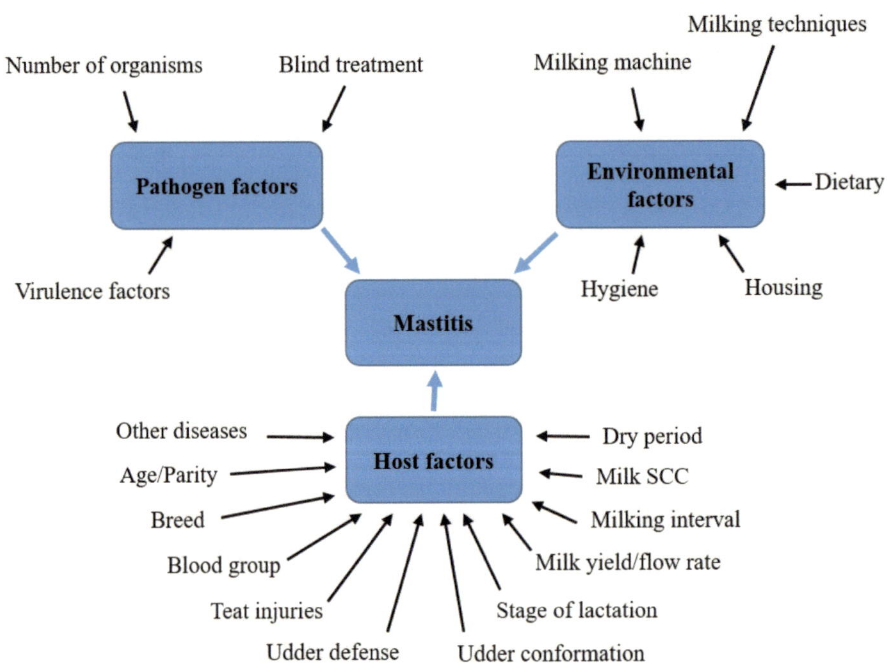

Figure 1.
Factors promoting mastitis. Source: Zigo et al. [3].

viruses, mycoplasma, yeasts, and algae, but bacteria have been identified as the principal causative agent of mastitis (95% of all IMI). In general, each mastitis case is believed to be caused by one primary pathogen, as in milk samples from the affected udder usually only one bacterial species has been identified. However, it is not rare to detect simultaneous infections by two different pathogen species, and even three pathogens have been found in a small proportion of samples [8, 9].

Major and minor pathogens are two main categories used to classify the microorganisms that cause mastitis. *Staphylococcus aureus, Streptococcus agalactiae*, or *Streptococcus dysgalactiale* are the most prevalent major pathogens or contagious udder pathogens, and when they can survive, these areas serve as their primary reservoirs in addition to the mammary gland (MG), the rumen, and the genital regions. As a result, the infection can spread from infected to uninfected quarters or halves [7]. Other pathogens that can cause intramammary infection in ruminants include *coliforms, enterococci*, *Streptococcus* spp., *Pseudomonas aeruginosa*, *Mannheimia hemolytica, Corynebacteria,* CoNS, and fungi, though their prevalence varies depending on the environment [10–12]. The most significant udder pathogens in this group are *Streptococcus uberis* and *E. coli*, which each have a number of pathogenic strains for both people and animals. Both pathogens can be present in the environment and the surroundings of the animals [7].

According to Slovak studies [7, 9, 13], *Staphylococcus chromogenes*, *Staphylococcus epidermidis*, and *Staphylococcus xylosus* are the most common pathogens from CoNS causing mastitis, followed by *Streptococcus agalactiae*, *Staphylococcus aureus*, *Streptococcus dysgalactiae*, *Escherichia coli,* and Enterococci. Of the 42 monitored dairy farms, CoNS and *S. aureus* accounted for 36% and 12% of all positive mastitic cases, respectively.

Namely, *S. aureus* and CoNS have been among the most common microorganisms causing mastitis in dairy cows and health disorders among consumers of milk and dairy products in recent years. According to the World Health Organization, 420,000 lives are lost due to food poisoning; and *Staphylococcus* spp. is characterized as an important agent that can cause foodborne diseases. Poisoning occurs due to the ingestion of preformed enterotoxins in food. Symptoms include vomiting, diarrhea, and cramps; and an outbreak could lead to a public health problem [12–14].

The MG's inflammatory process manifests as symptoms and modifications in the milk and udder tissue. The IMI can be categorized as either persistent (chronic) mastitis or subclinical mastitis. Subclinical forms, which do not exhibit overt indications of inflammation but instead have elevated somatic cell counts (SCC) in the presence of the causative agents, are typically a serious silent issue and are the most common illnesses to result in significant financial loss for owners. Since they cannot be detected without a lab or field test, the subclinical types of IMI frequently become incurable in later stages [9].

Staphylococci can induce different types of intramammary infections depending on the quantity and pathogenicity of the strains, as well as the degree of the udder tissue's response to damage or infection. The interaction between dairy animals' innate resistance and adaptive immunity, as well as the virulence of Staphylococcal strains, determines the course of the clinical inflammation of MG caused by Staphylococci, which is characterized by local visible inflammatory changes in milk and udder tissue, either with or without systemic clinical signs [15]. In general, if there are enough *S. aureus* penetrates into the teat, one of two clinical forms of IMI may develop. Peracute Staphylococcal mastitis occurs infrequently and primarily affects cows and ewes in early lactation with compromised immune systems. The illness is very severe, and is manifested by a high fever, depression, and inappetence. The animals may become comatose and die within

24 hours after the onset of symptoms. The reluctance of infected animals to move is related to grossly swollen infected quarters, which is extremely painful. Blood-stained secretion with serous fluid from the infected part of the udder is usually observed. In surviving animals, blue gangrenous patches may be observed on the infected udder tissue that progress to black, exuding sores [16]. Although early treatment with effective ATB can save an animal suffering from peracute *S. aureus,* the affected quarter is almost always lost [14].

The more common form of *S. aureus* infection is less severe but chronic. The animals with chronic mastitis may not appear affected, and the infected part of the udder does not cause pain. No abnormalities may be observed in the milk. The main complications associated with the treatment of *S. aureus* infection include the fact that many strains can cause this disease and increasing number of them are becoming resistant to an increasing range of antibiotics available for veterinary use. One of the frequent causes of growing resistance is the normal practice on farms of drying dairy cows universally with antibiotics in addition to treating clinical cases of IMI.

According to the study by Ferroni et al. [17] management practices are associated with increased antibiotic consumption, especially in intensive dairy production. The authors analyzed 101 beef and dairy cattle farms in central Italy and compared the overall average antibiotic consumption during one year. The total course of administered ATBs was 3 times higher in the case of dairy cows than in beef farms. Their increased number was mainly related to the treatment of lactating and drying cows with ATBs (**Figure 2**).

The studies Vasiľ et al. [18] and Holko et al. [19] confirm the increased resistance of mainly udder pathogens (*S. aureus, S. uberis, and S. agalactiae)* as well as CoNS to those ATBs, that are part of intramammary applicators used for dry treating.

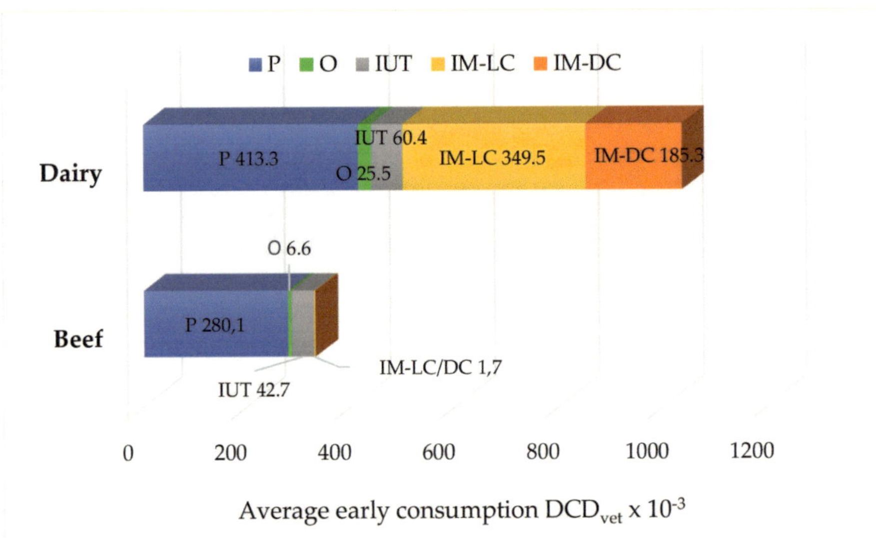

Figure 2.
Comparison of average early ATBs consumption between dairy and beef cattle.
Note: P = parenteral application, O = oral application, IUT = intrauterine application, IM-LC = intramammary treatment of lactating cows, IM-DC = intramammary application for drying). The overall average antibiotic consumption was expressed in defined course doses (DCD_{vet})/year and is presented per livestock specialization and by administration route. The total courses administered were higher in farms with intensive dairy production (1034.1×10^{-3} DCD_{vet}/year) than in beef farms (330.7×10^{-3} DCD_{vet}/year).

Lately, CoNS have become a concern among dairy producers, as their potential as mastitis-pathogens has been observed; and they have already been found in majority of other pathogens. Their predominant isolation can be explained by the fact that CoNS are pathogens adapted to survive in cows or ewes and may be in the mammary gland of sick or healthy animals; while some species are also more resistant to antibiotics than *S. aureus* [13]. Among all the CoNS found in dairy animals, *S. haemolyticus*, *S. chromogenes, S. epidermidis, S. warneri, S. cohnii, S. simulans, S. hominis, S.capitis, and S. xylosus* are the most prevalent species [20, 21].

Following a decline in the incidence of mastitis brought on by the infectious bacteria, the causative CoNS became more prevalent and more resistant to typical ATBs and disinfectants used in dairy farm conditions (**Table 1**). When compared to *S. aureus*, the CoNS often exhibits less virulence and pathogenicity. Their primary pathogenicity factors are biofilm formation and ATB resistance, which enable them to survive the use of medicines and disinfectants during therapy. In a study by Nascimento et al. [20], the most popular antimicrobials used in veterinary practice were tested in vitro against CoNS isolated from mastitic cows. High resistance to the ATBs used to treat cows during lactation was found in tested strains of *S. epidermidis*, *S. saprophyticus*, *S. hominis*, and *S. aerletae*. Also, they could also make some of the Staphylococcal enterotoxins.

Particularly, Staphylococci bacteria that are multiresistant to multiple ATBs pose a severe threat to the public's health [16]. Recent research also suggests that the presence of methicillin-resistant Staphylococci (MRS), which have been found in raw milk and dairyproducts, such as cheese, is indicated by multiresistant Staphylococci, particularly to *β*-lactam ATBs. The public's health is threatened, according to WHO, by

Number of resistant CoNS	Antimicrobial groups	Percentage of resistant strains	Source
16/37	Oxacillin + chloramphenicol	5.4%	Khazandi et al. [22]
	Oxacillin + novobiocin	27.0%	
	Oxacillin + tetracycline	5.4%	
	Oxacillin + cefoxitin	5.4%	
3/8	Ampicillin + clindamycin + oxacillin erytromycin + gentamycin + penicillin + sulfonamide + trimethoprim/sulfamethoxazole + tetracycline	37.5%	Dorneles et al. [23]
2/8	Ampicillin + penicillin + trimethoprim/sulfamethoxazole + trimethoprim/sulfamethoxazole	25.0%	
1/8	Ampicillin + gentamycin + oxacillin + penicillin + sulfonamide + trimethoprim/sulfamethoxazole + tetracycline	12.5%	
2/8	Ampicillin + gentamycin + oxacillin + penicillin + trimethoprim/sulfamethoxazole + tetracycline	25.0%	
18/170	Same group of antibiotics (*β*-lactam or MLS compounds)	10.58%	Sampimon et al. [24]
18/170	Diferent groups	10.58%	

Note: Number of resistant coagulase-negative staphylococci (CoNS); Antimicrobial groups they have resistance to; Percentage of resistant strains for each drug or group.

Table 1.
Resistance of CoNS to two or more antimicrobials.

the MRS strains' opportunistic capacity to induce mastitis. They might spread zoonotic diseases while acting as a gene repository for dairy cows' antimicrobial resistance. Of the MRS of concern, *Staphylococcus aureus* (MRSA) is the species most widely reported, however, in a number of studies CoNS were also identified as MRS isolates [23, 25, 26].

In addition to the increased antibiotic resistance of Staphylococci, the authors, Vasil et al. [18] and Haveri et al. [27] confirmed biofilm formation and lysines in mastitic milk samples and considered them as important virulence factors involved in the development of CM. Previous research has linked Staphylococci and their virulence factors to the pathogenesis and clinical manifestations of mastitis. They stressed the importance of thorough knowledge of their virulence factors, structures, and products. It is crucial to understand how these microorganisms facilitate adhesion and colonization of the mammary gland epithelium, which allows them to survive, successfully establish themselves, and persist in the host tissue. Therefore, the study was aimed at the occurrence and determination of contagious and environmental udder pathogens in dairy cows' and ewes' herds. Particularly in isolated Staphylococci, the presence of selected virulence factors such as hemolysis, gelatinase, biofilm, hydrolyzed DNA, and resistance to antibiotics with the detection of methicillin resistance gene-*mecA* and their effect on the severity of mastitis were determined.

2. Materials and methods

2.1 Monitored dairy farms

The practical part of the study was carried out in four different cows' and four sheep herds located in east Slovakia with conventional (nonorganic) farming. The selection of dairy farms for the study was based on criteria such as herd size, breed representation, and milk yield per lactation. Up to 70% of farms located in the east of Slovakia are in the range of 150–300 cattle and 200–400 ewes. Due to the study carried out in Slovakia, dairy farms were selected where there are national breeds of cattle and sheep. The practical part of the study on selected dairy farms with the clinical examination and collection of milk samples were approved by the Ethics Committee at the University of Veterinary Medicine and Pharmacy in Košice no. EKVP 2022/05.

From dairy cows, each herd size ranged from 150 to 300 Slovak spotted cattle bred between 1st and 4th lactation. The dairy cows under investigation on each of the four farms were housed in a system of free housing on straw litter with *ad libitum* access to water. According to international guidelines, a total mixed feed made up of silage, hay, and concentrate was given to them [28]. The rations met the nutritional requirements of cows weighing 650 kg, with an average milk yield of 20–30 kg per day. In the first phase of lactation, the mean average dry matter intake per cow per day was 23.6 kg +/- 3.7 kg. All cows were milked twice daily in parallel (Boumatic, USA) or fishing (DeLaval, Sweden) parlor. From all monitored dairy farms, 270 cows from the first, 215 cows from the second, 250 cows from the third and 225 cows from the fourth herd were investigated.

The four sheep farms were in herd sizes ranging from 200 to 400 animals and consisted of Improved Valachian, Tsigai, and Lacaune breeds. In April, the ewes were on pasture during the day and received concentrates in amounts of 200 g per day during milking. After their lambs were weaned in early April, the ewes were milked twice a day on each farm. In the first two herds, machine milking was performed using a two-line milk parlor 2×14 Miele Melktechnik, (Hochreiter Landtechnik, Germany) and in two other herds, the sheep were milked in two-line milk parlor 2× 16 Alfa Laval Agri

(Alfa Laval, Sweden). From all the monitored sheep farms, during the first month of pasture (April), 220 ewes from the first, 250 ewes from the second, 270 ewes from the third, and 200 ewes from the fourth herd were investigated.

2.2 Dairy animals selection and udder health examination

The dairy cows from four monitored farms were selected on the basis of the formation of production groups according to the stage of lactation (early lactation 14–100 days of lactation) and the phase of nutrition, which were compiled by the zootechnicians. The selected dairy cows of the same performance class (early lactation) were housed in individual husbandry groups, which included 45–90 animals on each farm.

Ewes from four herds were included in the study two months after lambing between the 1st and 3rd lactation with a stay on pasture and milked twice a day. Complex examination of health status of udder in ewes from four monitored farms was carried out at the start of the milking season (April). On the basis of a clinical assessment, each dairy cow and sheep had a thorough inspection that included sensory evaluation and udder palpation. The California mastitis test (CMT) (Indirect Diagnostic Test, Krause, Denmark) was used to evaluate the milk from the fore-stripping of each udder quarter or halve – Raw milk samples from cows and ewes with positive test results were collected [19]. CMT scores were 0, +, ++ and +++ for "negative", "weak positive", "positive" or "strong positive", respectively [29].

Following that, of the 960 cows that were investigated, 689 had a negative CMT score, and 271 cows had a CMT score that indicated trace or positive symptoms based on clinical manifestations (score of 1–3), were chosen for aseptic collection of 12 mL mixed quarter milk samples by discarding first squirts with the cleaning of the teat end with 70% alcohol for laboratory analyses of bacterial pathogens, according to Holko et al. [19]. From 940 examined ewes, 756 animals had negative CMT scores and 184 animals with CMT score trace or 1–3 were taken with 12 mL mixed halves milk samples for laboratory analyses. All milk samples from cows and ewes were cooled to 4°C and immediately transported to the laboratory and were analyzed on the following day.

According to the National Mastitis Council [30], each instance of mastitis in positive animals was given a grade that was divided into subclinical, clinical, and chronic forms. A high SCC was found utilizing a CMT evaluation and a positive bacteriological result to identify subclinical mastitis (SM), which was distinguished from clinical mastitis by the absence of obvious symptoms in the udder or alterations in the milk. Clinical mastitis (CM), which can be seen in the milk or in the udder, is divided into three stages: mild mastitis, which is identified by visible changes in secretion; moderate mastitis, which also exhibits localized MG inflammation; and severe mastitis, which also exhibits general symptoms like loss of appetite, difficulty standing, fever, or low body temperature. Based on repeated therapy, a history of clinical evaluation of the MG with a positive CMT score, and the development of udder pathogens, chronic mastitis, or persistent mastitis was identified.

2.3 Bacteriological culture and evaluation of growth on plates

In the laboratory, 0.2 mL of milk was inoculated from each sample onto a blood agar plate (Oxoid LTD, Hamshire, UK) and incubated aerobically at 37°C for 24 hours. The primocultivated colony from blood agar and identification of *Staphylococcus* spp. were sub-cultured onto different selective bacteriological media (No. 110, Baird-Parker agar, Brilliance UTI Clarity Agar, Oxoid, Hampshire, UK) and incubated at 37°C for next 24 hours. Cell morphology, Gram staining, the type of hemolysis, and the activities of catalase (3% H_2O_2, Merck, Darmstadt, Germany) were used to identify colonies, esculin hydrolysis and cytochrome oxidase C (Bactident Oxidase, Merck). The clumping factor test discovered potential *Staphylococcus aureus* (DiaMondiaL Staph Plus Kit, Germany). According to research by Vasil' et al. [18] and Holko et al. [19], esculin-positive streptococci were grown on modified Rambach agar to identify *Streptococcus uberis* or *Enterococcus* sp.. Lancefield serotyping (DiaMondiaL Strept Kit, Germany) was used to describe esculin-negative streptococci, and the MALDI-TOF MS (Bruker Daltonics, Bremen, Germany) was utilized to identify all gram-negative species. The presence of one or more colony-forming units (CFU) of the major udder pathogens, such as *Staphylococcus aureus, Streptococcus dysgalactiae, or Streptococcus agalactiae*, was considered positive. The sample would be deemed positive if the growth of a significant udder pathogen was discovered in conjunction with other environmental species. Other pathogens were categorized as requiring at least three CFUs to be present. If infectious pathogens did not develop and three or more pathogens were isolated from a single milk sample, the grown samples were deemed contaminated.

2.4 Detection of virulence factors in Staphylococci

Confirmed Staphylococci based on MALDI-TOF analysis were exposed to deoxyribonuclease (DNase test) and to produce extracellular proteolytic enzymes (Gelatin hydrolysis test) according to Hiko [31]. The formation of biofilm was determined by a phenotypic method by growth on Congo Red agar (CRA) according to Vasil' et al. [13].

Additionally, it was established that Staphylococci can generate hemolysins, based on Moraveji et al. [32]. After 24 and 48 hours of incubation at 37°C, the lysis zone of each Staphylococcal isolate on plates of blood agar base supplemented with 5% sheep blood was used to phenotypically define the different types of hemolysis.

The susceptibility of Staphylococci isolated from cows' (n = 136) and sheep's (n = 86) infected milk was tested *in vitro* against 14 antimicrobial agents. The susceptibility tests of isolates were carried out on Mueller Hinton agar using a standard disk diffusion procedure [33]. In the current study, antibiotic discs containing penicillin (PEN; 10 μg), ampicillin (AMP; 10 μg), amoxicillin (AMC; 10 μg), amoxicillin+clavulanic acid (AXC; 20/10 μg), ceftiofur (CEF; μg), oxacillin (OXA; 1 μg), cefoxitin (CFX; 30 μg), ciprofloxacin (CPR; 5μg). The diameters determined were classified as susceptible, moderate, or resistant based on CLSI breakpoints, and the zone of inhibition was measured in millimeters [34]. Reference strains of *S. aureus* CCM 4750 and *S. chromogenes* CCM 3386 from the Czech Collection of Microorganisms in Brno, Czech Republic, served as the controls in the assays. The study's chosen antimicrobials represent the range of medications used in veterinary care on Slovak dairy cows.

2.5 Detection of the mecA gene from Isolated Staphylococci

Phenotypical positive Staphylococci (45 and 26 isolates from cows' and sheeps' mastitic milk samples) based on their antimicrobial resistance to β-lactams antimicrobials were subjected to PCR to test for methicillin resistance. Total genomic DNA was isolated according to Hein et al. [35]. Using a BioSpec spectrophotometer, the purity of the DNA recovered from the tested Staphylococci was evaluated (Shimadzu, Japan). According to Poulsen et al. [36], acquired DNA was used in PCR reactions to detect the *mecA* gene using primers MecA1 and MecA2 (Amplia s.r.o., Bratislava, Slovakia). Sanger sequencing was used to confirm the identity of the PCR products (527 bp), in accordance with the guidelines provided by GATC Biotech (AG, Cologne, Germany). The BLAST tool was used to compare the DNA sequences acquired from the isolates to those found in the GenBank-EMBL (the European Molecular Biology Laboratory) database (NCBI software package). As a reference strain for PCR, *S. aureus* CCM 4750 (Czech Collection of Microorganisms, Brno, Czech Republic) was used in this investigation.

2.6 Statistical analysis

Microsoft Excel 2007® (Microsoft Corp., Redmond, USA) was used to process the study's data, and SPSS version 20 and Excel were used to analyze it (IBM Corp., Armonk, USA). According to specific microbial species and mastitis types, the findings of grown udder pathogens from mastitic cows and ewes were processed and converted to percentages. The percentage of resistant isolates from milk samples that tested positive for *S. aureus* and CoNS for each type of antibiotic was also used to express the antimicrobial resistance results. According to the production of virulence factors, Staphylococcal isolates from clinical, subclinical, or chronic mastitis were compared using the chi-squared test. The significance level was set at 0.05, the critical value $\chi 2$ was 2.206 for cows and 1.824 for ewes, and the testing value was G. Within each species, statistical independence between isolates with and without virulence factors was verified when $G > \chi 2$, although the independence was not statistically significant when assessing $G > \chi 2$.

3. Results

A thorough analysis of 960 dairy cows from four farms during the early lactation phase (14–100 days of lactation) revealed that 271 animals (28.2%) and 689 cows (71.8%), respectively, had CMT scores of trace or 1–3 for one or more quarters. 756 (80.4%) of the 940 ewes evaluated for udder health during the first month of the grazing season showed negative CMT results. One-hundred eighty-four ewes (19.6%) had positive CMT with a score trace of 1–3. Of the mixed milk samples taken from each examined cow and sheep based on the anamnesis and positive CMT score, bacterial agents causing a mastitis were identified in 230 (84.8%) and 155 (84.2%), respectively (**Figure 3**). For the presence of udder pathogens, 41 (15.1%) and 29 (15.7%) samples from examined cows and ewes with a positive CMT score were identified as negative or contaminated.

Based on the clinical examination of the MG, assessment of CMT, and laboratory diagnosis of milk samples, the occurrence of CM in the monitored cows' and sheep's dairy farms was 9.1% and 4.5%, respectively. The most common form of IMI in monitored cows and ewes was subclinical mastitis, with an incidence of 11.3% and 10.2%, respectively. The occurrence of chronic mastitis was 3.6% and 1.8% in monitored dairy cows and ewes, respectively. Of the cows' and ewes' positive samples, 136 and 86 cases (59.1% and 55.4% of the infected samples) contained the most commonly isolated Staphylococci, respectively (**Table 2**).

The CoNS represented the most commonly detected bacteria (42.6% and 39.9% of positive findings in cows and ewes), causing mainly subclinical mastitis. The *S. aureus* was the second most common pathogen (16.5% and 18.2% of positive findings in cows

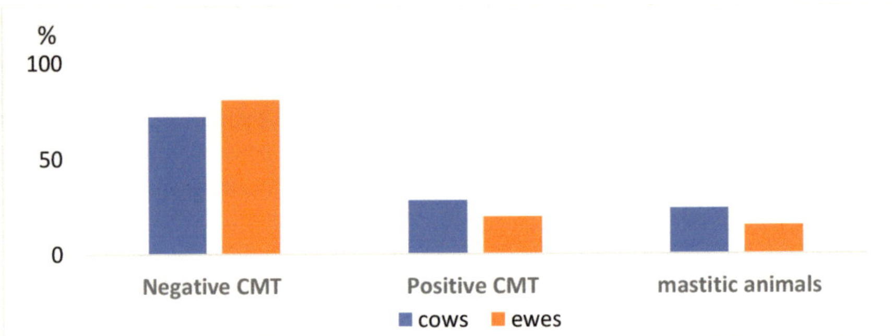

Figure 3.
Evaluation of CMT in monitored dairy herds.

and ewes, respectively), primarily causing clinical or chronic mastitis, followed by *E. coli*, streptococci, and enterococci (**Table 2**).

Tables 3 and **4** summarize, in descending frequency, the isolated strains of *Staphylococcus* spp., and indicate their role in the type of mastitis and the occurrence of selected virulence factors. Isolated *S. aureus* from clinical, chronic, or subclinical cases of mastitis has the highest ability to report virulence factors compared to CoNS and showed hemolysis in blood plates, production of gelatinase, biofilm, and the ability to hydrolyze DNA. The mecA gene was detected in two isolates of *S. aureus* from cows' clinical mastitis. Eight species of CoNS were isolated from mastitic cows, with the following recorded: *S. chromogenes* (22.4%), *S. warneri* (20.4%), *S. xylosus* (18.4%), *S. epidermidis* (9.1%), *S. haemolyticus* (7.1%), *S. hyicus* (10.2%), *S. capitis* (4.4%), and *S. piscifermentans* (4.4%) with testing value χ^2 = 2.206 for statistical significance. From mastitic ewes were isolated six species of CoNS with the following recorded: *S. warneri* (23.7%), *S. chromogenes* (18.6%), *S. xylosus* (18.6%), *S. haemolyticus* (15.2%), *S. caprae* (13.6%) and *S. epidermidis* (10.2%) with testing value χ^2 = 1.808 for statistical significance. From all the cows' and ewes' mastitic samples caused

Pathogens	Cows	Ewes	Clinical[1] n/%		Subclinical n/%		Chronic n/%	
	n/%	n/%	cows	ewes	cows	ewes	cows	ewes
CoNS	**98**/42.6	**59**/39.9	37/16	9/6.1	53/23.0	44/29.7	8/3.5	6/4.1
S. aureus	**38**/16.5	**27**/18.2	18/7.8	11/7.4	9/3.9	9/6.1	11/4.7	6/4.1
Escherichia coli	**26**/11.2	**18**/12.2	7/3.0	7/4.7	17/7.4	10/6.7	2/0.9	1/0.7
Str. uberis	**21**/9.1	**0**/0	9/3.9	0/0	5/2.2	0/0	7/3.0	0/0
Str. agalactiae	**8**/3.4	**4**/2.7	3/1.3	4/2.7	2/0.9	0/0	3/1.3	0/0
Streptococcus spp.	**10**/4.3	**9**/6.0	4/1.7	1/0.7	6/2.6	6/4.1	0/0	2/1.4
Enterococcus spp.	**14**/6.1	**24**/16.2	3/1.3	5/3.4	11/4.8	17/1.5	0/0	2/1.4
Mixed infection	**15**/6.5	7/4.7	6/2.6	5/3.4	5/2.2	10/6.7	4/1.7	0/0
Total	**230**/100	**155**/100	**87**/37.8	**42**/27.1	**108**/46.9	**96**/62.0	**35**/15.2	**17**/11.0

Clinical IMI[1] - clinical mastitis represented in mild, moderate, or severe forms of intramammary infection; n – number of mastitic animals. Modified from Zigo et al [9].

Table 2.
Pathogens isolated from milk samples of four monitored dairy cows and four sheep herds.

Staphylococcus spp./number	IMI[1]/number	Hemolysins[2]	DNAse[3]	Gelatinase	Biofilm	*mecA* gene	Testing value
S. aureus (38)	clinical (22)	6α/4δ/1β	14	17	9	2	5.447*
	chronic (8)	3α/2δ/2β	8	7	7	0	
	subclinical (8)	3α/1β	6	7	5	0	
Coagulase-negative Staphylococci with significant production of virulence factors							
S. chromogenes (22)	clinical (11)	4β/3δ	3	4	4	0	3.204*
	chronic (4)	3β	1	1	2	1	
	subclinical (7)	2β/2δ	1	1	2	0	
S. warneri (20)	clinical (9)	4δ/2β	2	2	4	1	2.688*
	chronic (3)	3β	0	0	1	0	
	subclinical (8)	3β/1δ	2	0	2	0	
S. xylosus (18)	clinical (7)	2δ/2β	2	0	3	0	2.255*
	chronic (1)	0	0	0	0	0	
	subclinical (10)	4β/1δ	0	0	2	0	
Coagulase-negative Staphylococci without significant production of virulence factors							
S. epidermidis (9)	clinical (2)	1δ	0	0	1	0	1.012
	subclinical (7)	2δ	0	0	2	0	
S. haemolyticus (7)	clinical (4)	2β/1δ	1	0	2	0	0.742
	subclinical (3)	0	0	0	0	0	
S. capitis (6)	clinical (2)	2δ	0	0	0	0	0.401
	subclinical (4)	0	0	0	0	0	
S. piscifermentans (6)	clinical (2)	1β	0	0	1	0	0.851
	subclinical (4)	2δ	0	0	0	0	
S. hyicus (10)	clinical (0)	0	0	0	0	0	0.332
	subclinical (10)	1δ	0	0	1	0	

*Legend: IMI[1]: the number of isolates and their impact on the type of mastitis; hemolysins[2]: the production of hemolysin type α, β or δ; DNAse[3]: the capability of Staphylococci to hydrolyze DNA; *Chi-squared test significance level α= 0.05; critical value χ^2 = 2.206. In isolated Staphylococci, Testing value (G) and statistical independence of virulence factors were validated when G > χ^2; the independence was not statistically significant when G < χ^2. Modified from Zigo et al. [9].*

Table 3.
*The role of **S. aureus** and CoNS in the form of mastitis from infected cows and their virulence factors.*

by CoNS, 48 and 26 (48.9% and 44.1%) cases involved the production of hemolysins, 12 and 11 (12.2% and 18.6%) the hydrolysis of DNA, 8 and 12 (8.1% and 20.3%) the production of gelatinase, as well as 27 and 14 (27.5% and 23.7%) involved biofilm production.

In **Table 3**, the significance level of α = 0.05 was confirmed in the isolated Staphylococci *S. aureus, S. chromogenes, S. warner*, and *S. xylosus* from CM and chronic cows' mastitis, which, when compared to less virulent strains, has the highest representation of virulence factors (production of hemolysins, gelatinase, the ability to hydrolyze DNA, and biofilm). In addition, the *mecA* gene was confirmed in one chronic case of mastitis in *S. chromogenes* and one CM case in *S. warneri*. In isolated

Staphylococcus *spp.*/number	**IMI[1]/number**	**Hemolysins[2]**	**DNAse[3]**	**Gelatinase**	**Biofilm**	***mecA* gene**	**Testing value**
S. aureus (27)	clinical (11)	4α/2δ/2β	6	9	4	0	3.288*
	chronic (6)	2α/1β	3	6	4	0	
	subclinical (10)	4α/2β	4	8	3	0	
Coagulase-negative Staphylococci with significant production of virulence factors							
S. warneri (14)	clinical (3)	1α/1β	1	2	2	0	2.305*
	chronic (3)	2β	1	1	1	0	
	subclinical (8)	2α/2β/	3	4	3	0	
S. chromogenes (11)	clinical (2)	1β	0	0	1	0	1.824*
	chronic (2)	1β	1	1	1	0	
	subclinical (7)	3β/1δ	3	2	2	0	
Coagulase-negative Staphylococci without significant production of virulence factors							
S. xylosus (11)	clinical (1)	1β	1	0	0	0	1.140
	subclinical (10)	4α/2β	2	2	2	0	
S. haemolyticus (9)	clinical (2)	1β	0	0	0	0	0.435
	chronic (1)	0	0	0	1	0	
	subclinical (6)	3β	0	0	0	0	
S. caprae (8)	clinical (1)	1β	0	0	0	0	0.341
	subclinical (6)	0	0	0	0	0	
S. epidermidis (6)	subclinical (7)	0	0	0	1	0	0.215

*Legend: IMI[1] - number of isolates and their influence on type of mastitis; hemolysins[2] - production of hemolysin type α, β or δ; DNAse[3] - ability of Staphylococci to hydrolyze DNA; *Chi-squared test significance level α = 0.05; critical value* $\chi^2 = 1.808$*; Testing value (G) and statistical independence of virulence factors in isolated Staphylococci was confirmed when* $G > \chi^2$*; the independence was not statistically significant when the testing value was* $G < \chi^2$*.*

Table 4.
*The role of **S. aureus** and NAS in the form of mastitis from infected ewes and their virulence factors.*

Staphylococci from mastitic ewes as demostrated in **Table 4**, the significance level in *S. aureus, S. warneri*, *S. chromogenes,* and *S. xylosus* was confirmed. The presence of the *mecA* gene has not been confirmed in tested *S. aureus* and CoNS.

In 136 and 86 isolates of Staphylococci from mastitic cows' and ewes' milk samples, *in vitro* resistance to 14 antimicrobials was tested by the standard disk diffusion method (**Table 5**). Generally, low resistance was shown to tetracycline, amoxicillin reinforced with clavulanic acid, rifaximin, and cephalexin. Of the tested Staphylococci, 95 and 38 isolates (70.0% and 44.2%) from mastitic cows and ewes showed resistance to one or more antimicrobials. To one antimicrobial, 50 and 22 isolates (36.7% and 25.6%) from mastitic cows and ewes were resistant. Mastitic cows and ewes produced 55 and 16 (39.7% and 18.6%) resistant Staphylococci isolates, respectively. Multidrug resistance to three or more antimicrobial classes was recorded in 16 and 4 isolates (11.7% and 4.7%) from cows' and ewes' samples. Tested Staphylococci showed multiresistance to a combination of antimicrobial classes, such as aminoglycosides, *β*-lactams, macrolides, and cephalosporins.

Number groups of antimicrobials	Phenotypic resistance profile	Cows (n = 136)		Ewes (n = 86)	
		No. of isolates	% of isolates	No. of isolates	% of isolates
0		41	30.1	48	55.9
1	PEN	7	5.1	4	4.7
1	STR	7	5.1	2	2.3
1	NMC	8	5.9	2	2.3
1	AMX	7	5.1	4	4.7
1	NVB	6	4.4	2	2.3
1	AMP	6	4.4	3	3.5
1	LNC	4	2.9	2	2.3
1	OXA	5	3.7	3	3.5
2	NMC, STR	8	5.9	2	2.3
2	OXA, NVB	0	0	2	2.3
2	OXA, TET	4	2.9	0	0
2	CPR, NVB	2	1.5	0	0
2	LNC, NVB	2	1.5	4	4.7
3	PEN, AMX, OXA	4	2.9	3	3.5
3	PEN, LNC, NVB	2	1.5	0	0
3	AMP, OXA, NMC	3	2.2	3	3.5
3	CPR, NMC, STR	4	2.9	0	0
3*	NVB, LNC, STR	4	2.9	2	2.3
4*	RFX, CPR, STR, TET	2	1.5	0	0
4*	CPR, LNC, NMC, NVB	3	2.2	1	1.2
4*	NVB, CPR, NMC, STR	2	1.5	0	0
4*	AMP, CEP, FOX, PEN	3	2.2	1	1.2
5*	OXA, AMP, LNC, NMC, STR	2	1.5	0	0
Total multidrug resistant isolates		16	11.8	4	4.7
Total antimicrobials resistant isolates		95	70.0	38	44.2

*Legend: *MDR: multidrug resistant isolates to three or more antimicrobial classes; AMX: amoxicillin, AMC: amoxicillin+clavulanat acid; AMP: ampicillin; CEP: cephalexin; CPR: ciprofloxacin; FOX: cefoxitin; LNC: lincomycin; NMC: neomycin; NVB:novobiocin; OXA: oxacillin; PEN:penicillin; RFX - rifaximin; STR:streptomycin; TET:tetracycline. Modified from Zigo et al. [9].*

Table 5.
*Phenotypic resistance profile in isolates of **Staphylococcus** spp. from mastitic cows and ewes.*

The 45 and 22 isolates (33.1% and 25.6% of all isolated Staphylococci) from mastitic cows and ewes in which phenotypic resistance was confirmed to β-lactam antimicrobials were tested by PCR for methicillin resistance with the detection of the *mecA* gene. From positive cows' milk samples, four isolates of Staphylococci - two of *S. aureus*, one of each of *S. chromogenes* and *S. warneri*, and one of each - were shown to contain the *mecA* gene and to be resistant to both cefoxitin and oxacillin. The outcomes of our research indicated that these isolates were methicillin-resistant Staphylococci (MRS).

4. Discussion

Milk and milk products are important global dietary products, consumed by more than 6 billion people worldwide. The recorded milk consumption in 2019 was 852 million tons, distinguishing the dairy industry as a very profitable market [1]. However, an infection of the mammary gland caused mainly by bacteria, mastitis, is still a major problem affecting animal welfare, productivity, and the economy; especially in dairy production, which can lead to losses for the dairy industry [37]. The incidence of mastitis is, of course, highly dependent on the lactation stage and health status of dairy animals [29, 38].

During the first 100 days of lactation, we observed the prevalence and etiology of mastitis in four dairy farms with cows and ewes. The majority of cows on the farms and the ones who produce the most milk are those that are in this early lactation stage (14–100 days after calving). The dairy cow produces an amount of milk during the first 100 days of lactation that accounts for 42–45% of the total milk. Aside from hormonal changes, decreased feed intake (which is in contrast to increased milk production), increased lipomobilization with a negative energy balance, and changes in body condition score, cows are also subject to stress factors as a result of this heavy milk production burden [38].

All of the aforementioned risk factors have an impact on both the non-specific and specific immune systems, specifically the MG, via which pathogenic microorganisms from the environment can enter the body more easily. An elevated SCC is one sign of the start of intramammary infection [39]. The qualitative test used in practice to detect mastitis is CMT, which reflects changes in milk consistency and SCC. Based on anamnesis, evaluation of CMT and clinical examination 689 (71.7%) of the 960 examined dairy cows were negative while 271 cows (28.2) showed positive, with scores from 1 to 3, or trace CMT. 230 (84.9%) of 271 cows showing high SCC were positive for the isolation of udder pathogens. This constitutes a significant risk for individual and herd health due to the high risk of spreading the infection to the environment. On monitored sheep's farms during the first month of pasture season, 756 sheep (80.4%) a negative CMT and 184 animals (19.6%) had increased SCC on the basis of CMT score (**Figure 1**). Laboratory examination revealed that 136 samples (14.5%) were positive for the presence of an udder pathogen.

The development of infection often starts when pathogens enter the duct system, travel via the teat canal, interact with the mammary tissue, multiply, and spread throughout the functioning parts of the udder, such as the milk cisterns. The degree to which the udder tissue reacts to injury or infection largely determines how mastitis manifests [7]. The most clinical cases are manifested by increased body temperature, inappetence, redness, swelling, and/or painful udder and/or abnormal milk. In the subclinical forms that were most often confirmed in our study, there were no apparent clinical signs, but an increase in SCC was observed in milk. Of the 230 and 136 infected cows and ewes, 46.9% and 62.0% had subclinical, 37.8% and 27.1% had clinical, and 15.2% and 11.0% had chronic mastitis (**Table 2**).

The major economic and health issues caused by CM, according to Singha et al. [11], include decreased milk output, poorer milk quality, higher expenses for treatment, involuntary culling, early cow rejection, increased risk of antibiotic resistance, and decreased animal welfare. Therefore, in high-yield dairy cows, CM prevalence should be at its lowest level. Our results indicate that the prevalence of CM in monitored cows' dairy farms was 9.1% which is in contrast with the studies of Silva et al. [40] and Rahman et al. [10], who reported the prevalence of CM from 2.3% to 4.1% in lactating cows.

The incidence of mastitis in sheep farms is extremely variable. Fthenakis [41] found the occurrence of mastitis in sheep is between 4 and 50%. In our study, the incidence of mastitis at the beginning of the pasture season was 16.4% in monitored sheep herds, with the most frequently occurring subclinical form (11.5%). The occurrence of CM was 4.9%, which is considered an acceptable value. On the contrary, studies from British slaughterhouses reported a very high prevalence of CM, ranging from 13–50%. This suggests that CM, or chronic mastitis, is a major cause of the culling of ewes in the UK [42].

According to Wenz et al. [43] and our investigation, gram-positive bacteria (*Staphylococcus* spp. or *Streptococcus* spp.) are frequently the cause of CM in dairy ruminants. However, depending on the farm layout and cleanliness level, a significant number of cows and ewes with coliform mastitis develop bacteremia, and 20% of udder infections are brought on by gram-negative pathogens. This is in line with our findings, which showed that SM and CM brought on by *E. coli* accounted for 11.2% and 12.2%, respectively, of infections from all infected cows and ewes.

Pyörälä and Taponen [12] point to a much-increased risk of CM caused by *S. aureus* and CoNS in a Finnish investigation on the detection and etiology of mastitis, which was also confirmed in all monitored dairy herds. CoNS (42.6% and 39.9% of the 230 and 155 infected cows and sheep samples, respectively) and *S. aureus* (16.5% and 18.2%), which were found in 136 and 86 cases, respectively (59.1% and 55.5%), were the most frequently found. In the milk samples from mastitic cows and ewes, the isolates of *S. aureus* and CoNS of the CM were responsible for 7.8% and 7.4%, and 16.0% and 6.1%, respectively. However, due to ongoing IMI, *S. aureus*, *S. chromogenes*, *S. warneri*, and *S. xylosus* frequently caused chronic mastitis. According to the findings of our investigation, studies by Holko et al. [19] and Idriss et al. [25] found a similar incidence of clinical and chronic mastitis caused by *S. aureus* and certain CoNS in the investigated dairy farms. More than half of all clinical and chronic IMI were caused by Staphylococci occurring more frequently than other udder pathogens (**Table 2**).

Chronic IMI rather than new infections are assumed as suggested by Persson et al. [44]. It has been reported that cows and ewes showing IMI in early lactation stage were also positive during the previous lactation or when dried off. These can originate a persistent subclinical infection into a chronic mastitis in animals that turn immunocompromised after calving or lambing.

Our findings are consistent with Holko et al. investigation's [19], which found a significant incidence of Staphylococci (CoNS and *S. aureus*) identified from tainted milk samples from 42 dairy farms in western Slovakia. The most often found bacteria was the CoNS, which made up 35.9% of positive samples. In contrast to our findings, the authors also confirmed high resistance to aminoglycosides and β-lactam antimicrobials without the presence of methicillin resistance genes. The dominant CoNS strains identified from mastitis in dairy ruminants in recent years, according to many reports, are *S. haemolyticus*, *S. chromogenes*, *S. warneri*, and *S. xylosus* [45–47]. CoNS has been mainly isolated from CM in addition to subclinical forms of IMI [45], which was validated in our investigation. CoNS-induced CM mastitis was associated with increased SCC, biofilm formation ability, and resistance to aminoglycosides and β-lactam antimicrobials, particularly penicillin, amoxicillin, and oxacillin.

The increasing prevalence of Staphylococcal infection in dairy ruminants is also influenced by the bacteria's level of pathogenicity and the production of certain virulence factors, which play a critical role in chronic and clinical mastitis cases [48, 49]. These contribute to the infection and include enterotoxins, different enzymes, and cell-associated factors. S. *aureus, S. chromogenes, S. warneri, S. xylosus*, and *S. haemolyticus* all produced hemolysins, hydrolyzed DNAse, and produced gelatinase from the various virulence factors. The isolated Staphylococci *S. aureus, S. chromogenes,* and *S. warneri* from mastitic cows and ewes had the most numerous representations of virulence factors, that may be contributing to the infection ability of isolated strains resulting in the increasing incidence of CM and persistent cases in comparison to strains with no virulence factors (**Tables 3** and **4**).

As biofilms promote Staphylococcal strains to adhere to both biotic and abiotic surfaces, they are regarded as having significant pathogenicity [48]. Bacteria generally produce a biofilm in order to protect themselves from fluctuations in environmental conditions. Substantial hygiene problems and economic losses are associated with biofilm formation in the dairy industry, as it can cause food spoilage and equipment impairment. The quality, quantity, and safety of food products are affected by the persistence of some foodborne pathogens on food contact surfaces and biofilms; and this problem has been reported more frequently [50]. Staphylococci are able to avoid immune defenses by creating biofilms that adhere to the MG epithelium, which leads to recurring or persistent infections [51]. Our findings indicated that seven species of NAS isolated from CM and chronic mastitis, as well as *S. aureus*, were mostly responsible for the biofilm-forming ability. The CoNS that produced chronic mastitis and CM showed the generation of hemolysins, the tendency to hydrolyze DNA, and resistance to antimicrobials as additional significant virulence factors in addition to *S. aureus*.

The relationship between hemolysins and biofilm formation, according to Perez et al. [49], can lessen the body's immunological response and response to antibiotic treatment while increasing Staphylococci interactions with bovine mammary epithelial cells. Our findings supported the idea that bacteria expressing these virulence characteristics had a high level of antibiotic resistance. In their study of Staphylococci isolated from mastitis milk in cows, Melchior et al. [51] indicated that the most frequent virulence factors in isolates recovered from CM were biofilm production and antibiotic resistance. Repeat episodes of mastitis following ineffective treatment showed increased biofilm production in CM strains. It is challenging to treat IMI brought on by *S. aureus* or CoNS even with intramammary antibiotics, therefore adequate care should be given to infections brought on by bacteria that produce biofilms.

The resistance to one or more antimicrobials in our study was detected in 95 and 38 isolates (77.0% and 44.2%) of Staphylococci isolated from infected cows and ewes, respectively. Multiresistant isolates for three or more groups of antimicrobial classes represented 16 and 4 isolates (11.8% and 4.7%). Multirresistance of staphylococci to a wide range of antibiotics such as β-lactams, macrolides, and cephalosporing (**Table 5**) was observed in our analysis. Methicillin resistance staphylococci were confirmed in 45 (33.1%) and 22 (25.6%) isolates from cows and ewes. By PCR the presence of the *mecA* gene was confirmed in two isolates of *S. aureus* and one isolate each of *S. chromogenes* and *S. warneri*, only from mastitic cows. Oxacillin and cefoxitin resistance was present in all *mecA*-positive Staphylococci (n = 4; 2.9%), and these strains were categorized as MRS. When the entire genome was sequenced for a research by Khazandi et al. [22], they discovered the presence of a *mecA* homolog in four oxacillin-resistant *S. sciuri* isolates. The homolog was not found using cefoxitin susceptibility testing or traditional *mecA* PCR. However, in our study, MRS was also phenotypically confirmed, so we do not assume the presence of a false positive *mecA* homolog.

The *S. aureus* and CoNS (n = 634; 36.7%) were the most frequently isolated bacteria from all tested samples in the study by Vyletelová et al. [52], which examined 1729 bulk milk and individual milk samples from ruminants in the Czech Republic. The species were also tested for the presence of the *mecA* gene using the PCR method and for antimicrobial susceptibility using the disc diffusion method. The most prevalent resistant strain was S. aureus (51%), followed by *S. epidermidis* (34.7%), and *S. chromogenes* (12.2%). A tital of 13 isolates of Staphylococci with β-lactam antibiotic resistance were found to have the mecA gene, which was primarily found in cow's milk. In a related investigation, Bogdanoviová et al. [53] tracked the prevalence and antibiotic resistance of *S. aureus* at 50 dairy farms in the Czech Republic. The authors found *S. aureus* positive in 58 samples from 261 raw milk and filtered milk samples, with 37 (14.2%) isolated from raw milk and 21 (8.1%) isolated from filtered milk. The majority of isolates from raw milk (17.8%) were found to be resistant to β-lactam antibiotics (amoxicillin and oxacillin), followed by isolates that were tetracycline- and macrolide-resistant. Methicillin-resistant *S. aureus* (MRSA) with the *mecA* gene present was found in two isolates from filtered milk and four isolates from raw milk samples using the PCR technique. We can affirm that IMI caused by Staphylococci, primarily *S. aureus*, with enhanced resistance to β-lactam antimicrobials is still a significant problem in Czech and Slovak dairy cow farms based on the findings of our study and the previous two investigations [52, 53]. The occurrence of MRS with the presence of the *mecA* gene is also worrying, which is in the range of 3–6% of isolates strains. In the monitored sheep, we did not record the presence of the *mecA* gene, which is probably a consequence of the higher culling of infected ewes with clinical and chronic mastitis and the renewal of herds with young sheep.

Among the resistant Staphylococci, *S. aureus* was identified by the WHO as the primary udder pathogen with the highest pathogenicity and most media attention. However, numerous other Staphylococci species have also been linked to methicillin resistance [54, 55]. In our work, we found the *mecA* gene to be present in two *S. aureus* isolates and one *S. chromogenes* and *S. warneri* strain. The CoNS is believed to be a reservoir for many resistance genes, which lead to greater resistance to antibiotics, according to Vinodkumar et al. [56]. The spread of resistance isolates may be caused, in part, by the presence of antimicrobials and their metabolites in the environment. This unfavorable effect of the heavy use of antimicrobials, along with delayed breakdown in the udder and drying out in cows (without antibiogram prior to application), maybe a contributing factor to rising resistance and MRS in veterinary medicine.

The MRS are usually resistant to β-lactam antimicrobials, and infections caused by these pathogens result in failed or frequent therapies, elevated SCC, and substandard milk quality. Studies from Norway revealed that MRSA has only ever been correlated to one case of cow mastitis when it comes to MRSA becoming the cause of the disease [23].

This contrasts with our findings and the current modeling in Belgium, where Bardiau et al. [56] revealed a comparable prevalence of MRSA in 4.4% of milk samples from clinical cases of mastitis and Vanderhaeghen et al. [57] identified MRSA in 9.3% of milk samples from farms relating with *S. aureus* mastitis, in contrast to our findings. Although our findings showed that the tested Staphylococci were more resistant to β-lactam antimicrobials than in previous studies, we can conclude that the occurrence of MRS in the monitored farms was roughly the same.

5. Conclusion

In dairy cows and ewes, Staphylococci and Streptococci were shown to be the most common causes of mastitis. Because of their virulence features, their prevalence poses a major risk to subsequent milk consumption. More than half of the mastitic cases from the cows and ewes under investigation were brought on by Staphylococci, particularly CoNS. Additionally, compared to other, less virulent CoNS strains, some strains of CoNS (*S. warneri, S. chromogenes*, and *S. xylosus*) with *S. aureus* isolated from clinical and chronic mastitis showed a high degree of pathogenicity in the synthesis of additional virulence factors. Resistance to aminoglycoside and β-lactam antimicrobials was frequently found in the tested Staphylococci, possibly because these are the antimicrobials most commonly used in dairy ruminant drying and mastitis treatment. Detection MRS by the presence of the *mecA* gene was confirmed in two isolates (2.9%) (one *S. aureus* and one isolate each of *S. chromogenes* and *S. warneri*) from mastitic cows. We can state that *S. aureus* still comes on top in the number of chronic or severe mastitis cases, as well as the number of virulence factors, but some CoNS species could have the same aggressive potential based on their production of gelatinase, hemolysis, biofilm, hydrolyzed DNA, and multidrug resistance.

According to the "*Farm to Fork*" strategy, the European Union intends to minimize the use of ATBs in cattle production by 50% by 2030 due to the frequent resistance of udder infections that cause mastitis and the occurrence of MRS in veterinary practice. Future use of antimicrobials during treatment in veterinary medicine and the dairy industry is still feasible, but only if it can be justified primarily in light of the findings of targeted diagnostics, which reveal each dairy animal's individual udder's physiological state through anamnestic data, clinical examination, SCC, and sample culture with an antibiogram. Designing effective prophylaxis and treatment guidelines to minimize the detrimental effects on milk yield and culling hazards in dairy animals requires knowledge of the virulence of both *S. aureus* and CoNS species associated with mastitis; particularly when combined with resistance patterns and the presence of MRS isolates.

Acknowledgements

The study was supported by Slovak grant **KEGA 009UVLF-4/2021**: *Innovation and implementation of new knowledge of scientific research and breeding practice to improve the teaching of foreign students in the subject of animal husbandry* and international **Visegrad Fund no. 22010056**: *Factors determining the occurrence of bovine mastitis in dairy herds situated in marginal regions.* The project is co-financed by the governments of Hungary, Poland, Czechia, and Slovakia through Visegrad Grants from the International Visegrad Fund.

Potential conflict of interest

The authors declare no conflict of interest.

Author details

František Zigo[1*], Zuzana Farkašová[1], Ibrahim Farag Mohammed Rehan[2,3] and Ahmed Sayed-Ahmed[4]

1 Department of Nutrition and Animal Husbandry, University of Veterinary Medicine and Pharmacy, Košice, Slovakia

2 Faculty of Veterinary Medicine, Department of Husbandry and Development of Animal Health, Menoufia University, Menoufia, Egypt

3 Faculty of Pharmacy, Department of Pathobiochemistry, Meijo University, Aichi, Japan

4 Faculty of Veterinary Medicine, Department of Anatomy and Embryology, Menoufia University, Menoufia, Egypt

*Address all correspondence to: frantisek.zigo@uvlf.sk

References

[1] FAO. Dairy market review, [Internet]. 2020. Available from: https://www.fao.org/3/cb2322en/CB2322EN.pdf

[2] Augère-Granier ML. The EU dairy sector: Main features, challenges and prospects. Briefing EU. [Internet]. 2018. Available from: https://www.europarl.europa.eu/thinktank/en/document/EPRS_BRI(2018)63034

[3] Zigo F, Vasil M, Ondrašovičová S, Výrostková J, Bujok J, Pecka-Kielb E. Maintaining optimal mammary gland health and prevention of mastitis. Frontier in Veterinary Science. 2021;**8**:607311

[4] Hogeveen H, Huijps K, Lam TJGM. Economic aspects of mastitis: New developments. New Zealand Veterinary Journal. 2011;**59**:16-23

[5] O'Kennedy R, Murphy C. Immunoassays: Development, Applications and Future Trends. 1st ed. New York, USA: Jenny Stanford Publishing; 2017

[6] van Soest FJS, Santman-Berends IMGA, Lam TJGM, Hogeveen H. Failure and preventive costs of mastitis on Dutch dairy farms. Journal of Dairy Science. 2016;**99**:8365-8374

[7] Cobirka M, Tančin V, Slama P. Epidemiology and classification of mastitis. Animals. 2020;**10**:1-17

[8] Dufour S, Labrie J, Jacques M. The mastitis pathogens culture collection. Microbiological Resources Announcement. 2019;**8**(15):e00133-e00119

[9] Zigo F, Farkašová Z, Výrostková J, Regecová I, Ondrašovičová S, Vargová M, et al. Dairy cows' udder pathogens and occurrence of virulence factors in Staphylococci. Animals. 2022;**4**:1-18

[10] Rahman M, Bhuiyan M, Kamal M, Shamsuddin M. Prevalence and risk factors of mastitis in dairy cows. Veterinary. 2010;**26**:54-60

[11] Singha S, Koop G, Persson Y, Hossain D, Scanlon L, Derks M, et al. Incidence, etiology, and risk factors of clinical mastitis in dairy cows under semi-tropical circumstances in Chattogram, Bangladesh. Animals. 2021;**11**:1-17

[12] Pyörälä S, Taponen S. Coagulase-negative Staphylococci - Emerging mastitis pathogens. Veterinary Microbiology. 2009;**134**:3-8

[13] Vasiľ M, Farkasova Z, Elecko J, Illek J, Zigo F. Comparison of biofilm formation by Staphylococcus aureus and Staphylococcus epidermidis strains isolated from sheep milk using three diagnostic methods. Polish Journal of Veterinary Sciences. 2017;**20**:795-801

[14] El-Diasty M, Talaat H, Atwa S, Elbaz E, Eissa M. Occurrence of Coagulase-negative Staphylococcal mastitis in dairy cows. Mansoura Veterinary Medical Journal. 2019;**23**:35-39

[15] Monistero V, Graber HU, Pollera C, Cremonesi P, et al. *Staphylococcus aureus* isolates from bovine mastitis in eight countries: Genotypes, detection of genes encoding different toxins and other virulence genes. Toxins (Basel). 2018;**10**(6):1-22

[16] Condas LAZ, De Buck J, Nobrega DB, Domonique AC, Roy JP, Greg PK, et al.

Distribution of non-aureus Staphylococci species in udder quarters with low and high somatic cell count, and clinical mastitis. Journal of Dairy Science. 2017;**100**:5613-5627

[17] Ferroni L, Lovito C, Scoccia E, Dalmonte G, Sargenti M, Pezzotti G, et al. Antibiotic consumption on dairy and beef cattle farms of central Italy based on paper registers. Antibiotics. 2020;**9**:1-23

[18] Vasiľ M, Elečko J, Zigo F, Farkašová Z. Occurrence of some pathogenity factors in coagulase negative Staphylococci isolated from mastitis milk in dairy cows. Potravinarstvo Slovak Journal of Food Science. 2012;**6**:60-63

[19] Holko I, Tančin V, Vršková M, Tvarožková K. Prevalence and antimicrobial susceptibility of udder pathogens isolated from dairy cows in Slovakia. The Journal of Dairy Research. 2019;**86**:436-439

[20] Nascimento JS, Fugundes PC, Brito AV, Dos Santos KR, Bastos MC. Production of bacteriocins by coagulase-negative Staphylococci involved in bovine mastitis. Veterinary Microbiology. 2005;**106**:61-71

[21] De Buck J, Ha V, Naushad S, Nobrega DB, Luby C, Middleton JR, et al. Non-aureus Staphylococci and bovine udder health: Current understanding and knowledge gaps. Frontiers in Veterinary Science. 2021;**8**:1-16

[22] Khazandi M, Al-Farha AAB, Coombs GW, O'Dea M, Pang S, Trott DJ, et al. Genomic characterization of coagulase-negative Staphylococci including methicillin-resistant Staphylococcus sciuri causing bovine mastitis. Veterinary Microbiology. 2018;**219**:17-22

[23] Fergestad ME, Visscher A, De L'Abee-Lund T, Ngassam TC, Mainil G, Thiry JD, et al. Antimicrobial resistance and virulence characteristics in 3 collections of Staphylococci from bovine milk samples. Journal of Dairy Science. 2021;**104**:10250-10267

[24] Sampimon OC, Lam TJGM, Mevius DJ, Schukken YH, Zadoks RN. Antimicrobial susceptibility of coagulase-negative Staphylococci isolated from bovine milk samples. Veterinary Microbiology. 2011;**50**:173-179

[25] Idriss SE, Foltys V, Tančin V, Kirchnerová K, Zaujec K. Mastitis pathogens in milk of dairy cows in Slovakia. Slovak Journal of Animal Science. 2013;**46**:115-119

[26] Dorneles EMS, Fonseca MDAM, Abreu JAP, Lage AP, Brito MAVP, Pereira CR, et al. Genetic diversity and antimicrobial resistance in *Staphylococcus aureus* and coagulase-negative Staphylococci isolates from bovine mastitis in Minas Gerais, Brazil. Microbiologyopen. 2019;**8**:1-7

[27] Haveri M, Roslöf A, Pyörälä S. Virulence genes of bovine Staphylococcus aureus from persistent and nonpersistent intramammary infections with different clinical characteristics. Journal of Applied Microbiology. 2007;**103**:993-1000

[28] NRC. Nutrient Requirements of Dairy Cattle. 7th ed. Washington, USA: The National Academies Press; 2001. p. 381

[29] Tančin V, Mikláš Š, Čobirka M, Uhrinčať M, Mačuhová L. Factors affecting raw milk quality of dairy cows under practical conditions. Slovak Journal of Food Science. 2020;**14**:744-749

[30] NMC. National Mastitis Council Recommended Mastitis Control Program. Verona, WI: Natl. Mastitis

Counc. Ann. Mtg. Proc., Reno, NV. Natl. Mastitis Counc., Inc; 2001. p. 408

[31] Hiko A. DNase-cross-Coagulase test and antimi-crobial resistance test on Staphylococcus along beef abattoir line in Addis Ababa Ethiopia. Ethiopia Veterinary Journal. 2019;**23**:90-110

[32] Moraveji Z, Tabatabaei M, Shirzad AH, Khoshbakht R. Characterization of hemolysins of Staphylococ-cus strains isolated from human and bovine, southern Iran. Iranian Journal of Veterinary Research. 2014;**15**:326-330

[33] CLSI document M2-A13. Performance standards for antimicrobial disk susceptibility tests, Thirteenth informa-tional supplement. Clinical and Laboratory Standards Institute, Wayne, PA, USA. 2018. p. 92

[34] CLSI document M100–S31. Performance standards for antimicrobial susceptibility testing; Thirty–first informa-tional supplement. Clinical and Laboratory Standards Institute, Wayne, PA, USA. 2021. p. 350

[35] Hein I, Jorgensen HJ, Loncarevic S, Wagner M. Quantification of Staphylococcus aureus in unpasteurised bovine and caprine milk by real-time PCR. Research in Microbiology. 2005;**156**:554-563

[36] Poulsen AB, Skov R, Pallesen LV. Detection of methicillin resistance in coagulase-negative Staphylococci and in Staphylococci directly from simulated blood cultures using the EVIGENE MRSA Detection Kit. The Journal of Antimicrobial Chemotherapy. 2003;**51**:419-421

[37] Abera A. Prevalence and associated risk factors of bovine mastitis in lactating cows of small holder dairy farms in Ethiopia. Journal of Veterinary Medicine and Surgery. 2020;**4**(2):1-7

[38] Nitz J, Wente N, Zhang Y, Klocke D, Seeth M, Krömker V. Dry period or early lactation-time of onset and associated risk factors for intramammary infections in dairy cows. Pathogens. 2021;**10**:1-19

[39] Tančin V. Somatic cell counts in milk of dairy cows under practical conditions. Slovak Journal of Animal Science. 2013;**46**:31-34

[40] Silva AC, Laven R, Benites NR. Risk factors associated with mastitis in smallholder dairy farms in Southeast Brazil. Animals. 2021;**11**:1-10

[41] Fthenakis GC. Prevalence and aetiology of subclinical mastitis in ewes of Southern Greece. Small Ruminant Research. 1994;**13**(3):293-300

[42] Conington J, Cao G, Stott A, Bünger L. Breeding for resistance to mastitis in United Kingdom sheep, a review and economic appraisal. The Veterinary Record. 2008;**162**(12):369-376

[43] Wenz JR, Barrington GM, Garry FB. Bacteremia associated with naturally occuring acute coliform mastitis in dairy cows. Journal of the American Veterinary Medical Association. 2001;**219**:976-981

[44] Persson WK, Bengtsson B, Lindberg A, Nyman A, Ericsson UH. Incidence of mastitis and bacterial findings at clinical mastitis in Swedish primiparous cows- influence of breed and stage of lactation. Veterinary Microbiology. 2009;**134**:89-94

[45] Supre K, Haesebrouck F, Zadoks RN, Vaneechoutte M, Piepers S, De Vliegher S. Some coagu-lase-negative Staphylococcus species affect udder health more than others. Journal of Dairy Science. 2011;**94**:2329-2340

[46] Hosseinzadeh S, Saei HD. Staphylococcal species associated with bovine mastitis in the North West of Iran: Emerging of coagulase-negative Staphylococci. International Journal of Veterinary Science and Medicine. 2014;**2**:27-34

[47] Zigo F, Elecko J, Vasil M, Ondrasovicova S, Farkasova Z, Malova J, et al. The occurrence of mastitis and its effect on the milk malondialdehyde concentrations and blood enzymatic antioxidants in dairy cows. Veterinary Medicine. 2019;**64**:423-432

[48] Fredheim EGA, Klingenberg C, Rodhe H, Frankenberger S, Gaustad P, Flaegstad T, et al. Biofilm formation by Staphylococcus haemolyticus. Journal of Clinical Microbiology. 2009;**47**:1172-1180

[49] Pérez VKC, Da Costa GM, Sá Guimarães A, Heinemann MB, Lage AP, Dorneles EMS. Relationship between virulence factors and antimicrobial resistance in Staphylococcus aureus from bovine mastitis. Journal of Global Research. 2020;**22**:792-802

[50] Shemesh M, Ostrov I. Role of Bacillus species in biofilm persistence and emerging antibiofilm strategies in the dairy industry. Journal of the Science of Food and Agriculture. 2020;**100**:2327-2336

[51] Melchior MB, Van Osch MHJ, Lam TJGM, Vernooij JCM, Gaastra W, Fink-Gremmels J. Extended biofilm susceptibility assay for Staphylococcus aureus bovine mastitis isolates: Evidence for association between genetic makeup and biofilm susceptibility. Journal of Dairy Science. 2011;**94**:5926-5937

[52] Vyleťelova M, Vlkova H, Manga I. Occurrence and characteristics of methicillin resistant Staphylococcus aureus and methicillin resistant coagulase-negative Staphylococci in raw milk manufacturing. Czech Journal of Food Sciences. 2011;**29**:11-16

[53] Bogdanovičová K, Skočková A, Šťástková Z, Karpíšková R. Occurrence and antimicrobial resistance of Staphylococcus aureus in bulk tank milk and milk filters. Slovak Journal of Food Science. 2014;**8**:97-101

[54] Seixas R, Santos JP, Bexiga R, Vilela CL, Oliveira M. Short communication: Antimicrobial resistance and virulence characterization of methicillin-resistant Staphylococci isolates from bovine mastitis cases in Portugal. Journal of Dairy Science. 2014;**97**:340-344

[55] Vinodkumar K, Neetha N, Ashok S, Suchithra S, Justin D, Radhik S. Genotypic and phenotypic *β*-lactam resistance and presence of PVL gene in Staphylococci from dry bovine udder. PLoS One. 2017;**12**:1-19

[56] Bardiau MK, Yamazaki JN, Duprez B, Taminiau J, Mainil G, Ote I. Genotypic and phenotypic characterization of methicillin-resistant *Staphylococcus aureus* (MRSA) isolated from milk of bovine mastitis. Letters in Applied Microbiology. 2013;**57**:181-186

[57] Vanderhaeghen W, Cerpentier T, Adriaensen C, Vicca J, Hermans K, Butaye P. Methicillin-resistant *Staphylococcus aureus* (MRSA) ST398 associated with clinical and subclinical mastitis in Belgian cows. Veterinary Microbiology. 2010;**144**:166-171

Section 4

New Treatments

Chapter 7

The Ability of Some Inorganic Nanoparticles to Inhibit Some *Staphylococcus* spp.

Abdalmohaimen Suood, Iman Mahdi and Mahmood Saleh

Abstract

In the last decades, antibiotics were used to treat infections caused by some *Staphylococcus* species, especially *Staphylococcus aureus* and *Staphylococcus epidermidis*. The widespread use of antibiotics to treat staphylococcal infections has resulted in an increase in the resistance of bacteria to antibiotics, particularly to beta-lactam antibiotics. In recent years, researchers have been working on developing new antibiotics, despite the fact that they are complex and expensive and carry a number of risks associated with drug toxicity. Using new substances that have good potential against bacterial infection without causing bacteria to become resistant to these substances is currently being researched. More research has been carried out on the effect of silver and copper nanoparticles in neutralizing staphylococcal infection in laboratory studies. The toxic effect of nanoparticles was a concern to scientists, but despite that, the studies *in vivo* found that there was no toxic effect at low doses of nanoparticles on rats. The findings in this field were acceptable to entice researchers to develop these substances.

Keywords: *Staphylococcus aureus*, *Staphylococcus epidermidis*, silver, copper, nanoparticles

1. Introduction

Bacteria belong to prokaryotic organisms, which means they have no clear nucleus such as in eukaryotic organisms. Many bacteria exist as normal flora in or on human skin, and some bacteria are opportunistic and pathogenic to their hosts; Staphylococcal bacteria have a large number of species. The species that are mentioned more than once in scientific reports that cause infections and pathogenicity to their hosts are *S. aureus* and *S. epidermidis* [1, 2]. *S. aureus* is Gram-positive bacteria that causes a variety of diseases. Furthermore, *S. epidermidis* has been identified as a second cause of wound inflammation after *S. aureus* in the last two decades [1]. Chemotherapy (antibiotics) and biological therapy have been used to eliminate the pathogenicity of some bacteria for decades.

Although some of the antibiotics have good results in reducing the pathogenicity of some Staphylococcal bacteria, the problem of resistance has begun to appear, for example, methicillin-resistant *S. aureus* (MRSA). A new agent has been applied to solve this problem, represented by nanomaterials. Silver and copper nanoparticles showed a nice result against selected pathogen isolates that were resistant to agents of antibiotics [3, 4].

This chapter explores a brief overview of *S. aureus* and *S. epidermidis,* as well as the impact of some nanoparticles in the suppression of their pathogenicity.

2. *S. aureus*

S. aureus produces a purple stain when Gram stain is applied to it, for this reason, it is named Gram-positive bacteria. This species is found mainly as part of the natural microbiota on the skin, gland skin, and infrequently in the mucous membrane of birds and mammals. *S. aureus* becomes more pathogenic than other Staphylococcal species, such as *S. epidermidis*, when suitable habitat elements are provided. *S. aureus*, which is cited in numerous scientific studies, causes a variety of diseases [5]. The virulence factors that make this species more ferocious against its host are the source of its illnesses. The use of antibiotics to treat pathogenic bacteria has increased over the last 10 years. Therefore, *S. aureus* has become increasingly resistant to antibiotics, as seen by the MRSA strain.

3. *S. epidermidis*

Another Gram-positive bacteria species is *S. epidermidis*. *S. epidermidis* belongs to coagulase-negative Staphylococci (CoNS), which means it lacks the enzyme coagulase, compared with *S. aureus*, which has the enzyme coagulase [6]. The usual inhabitant can also be found in human skin and mucosal membranes. *S. epidermidis* is infrequently known to cause infections in normal humans, but infections of this species are becoming more common in susceptible patients, particularly long-term hospital patients or patients with implanted foreign bodies [7, 8]. *S. epidermidis* has the ability to attach and develop on polymer surfaces, then produce extracellular slime substances, and finally cause the pathogenesis of polymer-associated illnesses [9]. The slime substance clearly guards the imbedded Staphylococci against antibiotics. Frígols et al. [10] have found that methicillin-resistant *S. epidermidis* (MRSE) is a common cause of infectious keratitis caused by *S. epidermidis* and shows a high rate of multidrug resistance.

4. Glance of nanotechnology

Nanotechnology is a new science with a short history of knowledge. Nanotechnology applications make revolutions in many fields because nanomaterial characterizations have a huge difference compared with bulk materials [11]. Bionanotechnology is a term used to describe a subfield of nanotechnology that deals with biology. It describes any materials or processes at the nanoscale that are based on biological or biologically inspired molecules, such as nanotechnology devices used in controling and monitoring in medicine. Another example uses nanocarriers loaded with medicine that are used to introduce therapy into pathogen microbes or unusual cells that belong to tissue (cancer therapy) [12]. Nanoparticles are incredibly tiny particles with sizes between 1 and 100 nanometers. Several nanoparticles have been used to test their activity against harmful microbes. Methods to synthesize these particles are divided into three categories, which are biological, chemical, and physical. Inorganic reducing agents are used in nanoparticle syntheses, such as silver and copper nitrate. Numerous inorganic nanoparticles have been employed in numerous scientific articles [13–15]. Among these, silver and copper nanoparticles are two that will be discussed in the subsections that follow.

4.1 Silver nanoparticles

Silver nanoparticles have attracted interest in the biological field due to their special characteristics, such as size and shape that depend on magnetic, optical, and electrical properties [16]. These characteristics also make it possible to use silver nanoparticles in antimicrobial applications and other medical-related applications. Many biological, chemical, and physical methods have been employed to synthesize and stabilize silver nanoparticles [17]. The popular methods for the production of nanoparticles are chemical approaches. The method using chemical materials almost contains toxic materials. Therefore, chemical methods are considered toxic, not eco-friendly, and expensive ways to synthesize nanoparticles. For this reason, easy and simple methods are required to produce silver nanoparticles without using harmful or expansive materials. Biological or green chemistry has been used in recent years in abundance [18]. Microorganisms or plant extracts are used as reducing agents to inorganic raw materials for nanoproducts [19, 20].

4.1.1 Silver nanoparticles with anti-pathogenic properties

The problem of resistant pathogen bacteria to antibiotics and the product of another generation of antibiotics is a big challenge to scientists at present. Development of a new generation of antibiotics takes time and is expansive. It is necessary to find another medicine that has stability with activity without resistant pathogen bacteria to it. It is necessary to treat harmful bacteria. Inorganic nanoparticles are a current drug that is hoped to be effective almost immediately. Silver nanoparticles have been widely used as antibacterial agents in the medical field, food storage, textile coatings, and a variety of environmental applications. Silver nanoparticles' antimicrobial qualities have led to their employment in a variety of disciplines including medicine, industry, animal husbandry, packaging, accessories, cosmetics, health, and military applications [21]. The interest in the activity of silver nanoparticles toward the pathogen *S. aureus* has increased in the last 8 years, as shown in **Figure 1**.

The study of the synergetic effect of silver nanoparticles with antibiotics, for example, erythromycin, amoxicillin, penicillin G, clindamycin, and vancomycin against *S. aureus* [23] was another hope. The technique approved its activity against pathogen bacteria *in vitro* (inside laboratory). Due to the perfect results of antibacterial activity of silver nanoparticles combined with some antibiotics *in vitro* assay, these results inspired the researchers to assay this technique *in vivo* tests using animal models (inside the organism's body) [24]. Xu et al. [25] demonstrated the effect of silver nanoparticles combined with vancomycin, rifampin, and other antibiotics used in their study *in vitro* as well as *in vivo* assay. The silver nanoparticles successfully passed assays *in vitro* and *in vivo* and hope to be used for human treatment in the next few years.

Resistance to silver nanoparticles by bacterial cells has been reported. Elbehiry et al. [26] explored the resistance development of *S. aureus* to silver nanoparticles

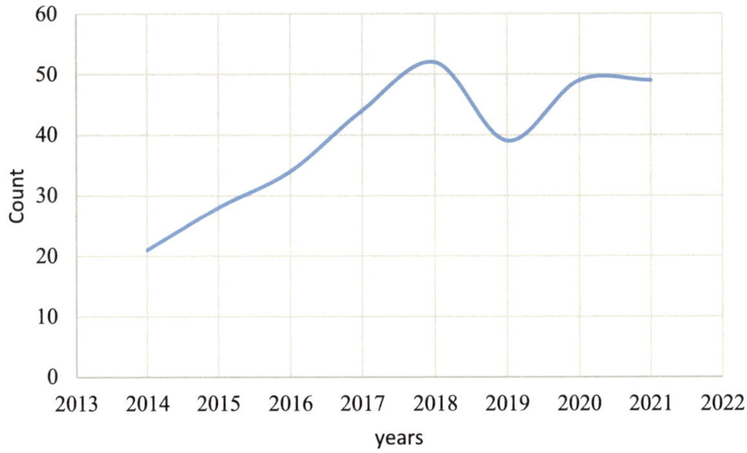

Figure 1.
Increasing publication regarding the activity of silver nanoparticles against the pathogen Staphylococcus aureus *in recent years [22].*

after multiple generations of *S. aureus*. As well, Panáek et al. [27] demonstrated that after repeated exposure to inhibitor concentrations of silver nanoparticles, Gram-negative bacteria such as *Escherichia coli* develop resistance to silver nanoparticles. This resistance is not concerning due to these phenotypic changes and not genetic changes, which means this factor will not be transported to future generations of bacteria cells. Furthermore, the multiple mechanisms of action of nanoparticles may limit the development of bacterial resistance to nanoparticles.

4.2 Copper nanoparticles

Finding another nanoparticle with excellent properties at a lower cost is becoming more required nowadays. Copper nanoparticles have been widely used as inexpensive and effective therapeutic for certain harmful bacteria. Therefore, copper nanoparticles could be a useful antibacterial agent in the coming days. Copper nanoparticles are highly reactive due to their high surface-to-volume ratio; this allows them to easily interact with other particles and boost their antibacterial efficiency. Copper nanoparticles have received much interest because of their unique physiochemical properties, surface-to-volume ratio, cheap preparation, and nontoxic preparation. They have many amazing uses in various domains, such as anticancer activity [28], antimicrobial activity [29], antifungal activity [30], catalysts [31], and antioxidant activity [32]. The creation of copper nanoparticles has been described in numerous scientific works using chemical, physical, and biological methods [33]. The biological method uses natural reducing agents that can be found in plant extracts, fungi, and bacteria to convert copper salt into copper nanoparticles [34–36]. A commendable job has been done regarding the production and stability of copper nanoparticles by using biological processes.

4.2.1 Copper nanoparticles as antibiotics for some human pathogen bacteria

Copper metal is one of the essential elements, especially in most living organisms. The particles of copper in the nanoscale have different properties compared with copper particles and have many applications, one of them is an antibacterial agent. Copper nanoparticles possess better properties as inorganic antibacterial agents relative to other expansive metal nanoparticles such as gold and silver [37]. For instance, the copper nanoparticles recorded higher antibacterial activity relative to silver nanoparticles against some human pathogen bacteria [38].

According to **Figure 2,** copper nanoparticles have received a lot of attention from researchers lately due to their antibacterial action against many pathogens of *S. aureus* [40].

Despite only a few scientific studies examining the efficacy of copper nanoparticles against *Staphylococcus epidermidis* [41, 42], they have revealed potency against this isolate. Consequently, it is a promising medical treatment.

Another strategy has been applied using a solution of antibiotics with copper nanoparticles. Selvarani [43] showed the effect of tetracycline alone against *S. aureus*, recording an inhibition zone at 25.3 mm using the disc diffusion method, but when impregnating the disc of antibiotics with 50 μl of freshly prepared copper nanoparticles, the diameter of the zone of inhibition was increased to 32.6 mm, increasing by 28%. The same study with another antibiotic (Rifampicin) recorded an increase of 13.8% compared with Rifampicin alone. Additionally, Woźniak-Budych et al. [44] investigated the activity of Rifampicin combined with copper nanoparticles toward four bacterial strains, one of those being *S. aureus*, and found a synergic effect of Rifampicin with nanoparticles was a successful way to prevent the development of resistance. Therefore, there is hope through combining inactive antibiotics with some inorganic copper nanoparticles to convert them into active antibiotics. It is another promising solution to the problem of *S. aureus* and *S. epidermidis* antibiotic resistance.

4.3 Mechanism of antibacterial activity of silver and copper nanoparticles toward bacteria

The antibiotics are categorized according to their specific targets, which makes them safe for human use. Antibiotics' mechanisms of action include five basic mechanisms against bacterial cells, which are inhibition of cell wall synthesis, inhibition of

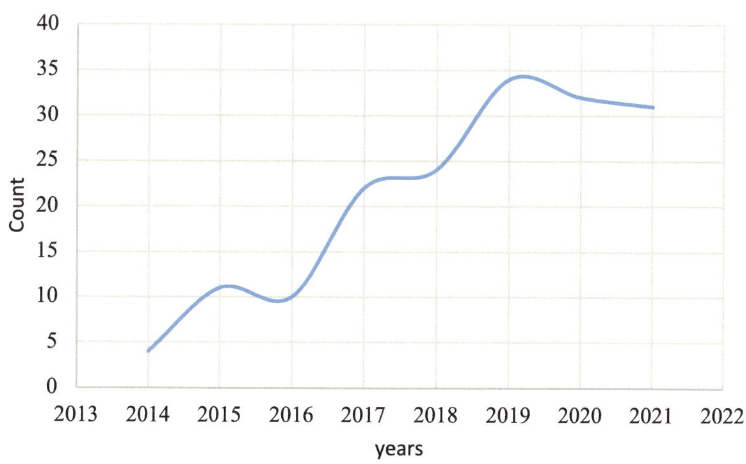

Figure 2.
Increasing publication regarding the activity of copper nanoparticles against the pathogen Staphylococcus aureus *in recent years [39].*

protein synthesis (translation), alteration of cell membranes, inhibition of nucleic acid synthesis, and finally antimetabolite activity [45]. Silver nanoparticles no longer have a clear mechanism, such as antibiotics against pathogenic bacteria, but many studies have been conducted on their possible mechanisms of antibacterial properties [46–48]. In recent years, silver nanoparticles have been used in many fields, including medicine, air and water purification, and others [49].

The properties of the mechanisms for silver nanoparticles are well described [48]. The nanoparticles of silver that adhere to the surface of the bacterial cell membrane probably disrupt the functions of the cell membrane, such as respiration and substance transport, as well as cell membrane separation from the cell wall partial or complete [50]. The increased stickiness of nanoparticles results in increased destruction permeability capacity and cell division that lead to a fast rate of death for bacteria compared with the low concertation of nanoparticles. The above description includes the hypothesis of silver nanoparticles' mechanism of antibacterial that sticks to cell walls and cell membranes. The silver nanoparticles can pass through the cell wall of bacteria and reach the cell membrane easily because there are pores in the cell wall. However, there is another hypothesis about silver nanoparticles that successfully reach inside bacterial cells. As a result, silver nanoparticles' creation links with phosphorus and sulfur present in cytoplasmic molecules of bacteria, such as DNA, causing the death and destruction of bacteria [51]. Another possible effect of silver nanoparticles is the disruption product of energy compounds (adenosine triphosphate ATP) and the generation of DNA. They then produce reactive oxygen species (ROS), which are considered toxic to bacterial cells [52].

The mode of action of copper nanoparticles toward antibacterial has little information explained. The researcher proposed the mechanism of activity of copper nanoparticles on pathogen bacteria may have a similar mode of action to silver nanoparticles [53]. Schrand et al. [54], it was hypothesized that copper nanoparticles work as antibacterial agents against many bacteria species due to interaction with SH-groups that result in protein denaturation. Copper nanoparticles may have an effect on cell membrane because of their affinity toward the amines and carboxyl groups that are found on the membranes of some bacteria strains [55]. The nanoparticles can enter a cell through the pores in the cell membrane because of their nanoscale size, or get inside bacteria through ion channels and transport proteins in the membrane of bacteria. After copper nanoparticles enter the cell, they may bind to DNA molecules and disturb the structure of the DNA strands, as well as find copper ions inside bacterial cells, which also disturb biochemical processes [56]. Deryabin et al. [57] hypothesized another mechanism, copper nanoparticles may accumulate on the cell of bacteria and diffuse inside the cell, causing oxidative stress that causes the cell of bacteria to die. **Figure 3** depicts all possible mechanisms of action for silver and copper nanoparticles. Due to limited studies discussing the mechanisms of bioactivities of copper nanoparticles against bacteria, the mechanism of action of copper nanoparticles needs more studies about their cytotoxicity and safety to be used as a human medicine agent to treat harmful bacteria.

4.4 The possible toxic effects of silver and copper nanoparticles

The toxic effects of nanoparticles of silver and copper have been studied. In the study by Nakkala et al. [58], the rats were treated orally with 5 and 10 mg/kg of silver nanoparticles for 28 days. The rat organs, such as liver, lungs, kidney, spleen, heart, testes, and brain, showed no histopathological changes at the end of the test. Elbehiry

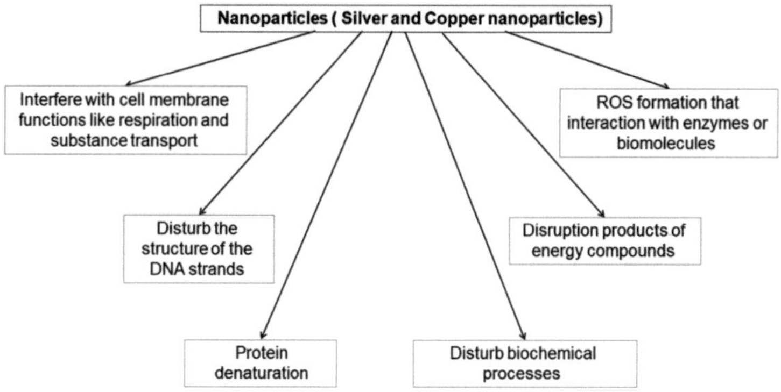

Figure 3.
Nanoparticles' possible mechanism of action on and in bacterial cells.

et al. [26] also studied the toxic effects of silver nanoparticles at 0.25, 0.5, and 1 mg/kg in the brain, liver, kidneys, heart, and spleen of rats. After 28 days of testing, they did not find any histological changes in the organs of experimental animals. In contrast with the findings of Kim et al. [59], they noted that after feeding the rat with silver nanoparticles for long-term oral administrated concentrations of 30, 300, and 1000 mg/kg, any changes in the weight of the rat body were not recorded, but they noted the accumulated silver nanoparticles in different tissue organs. In addition, Tiwari et al. [60] found that the treated cells of the liver and kidney with high doses of silver nanoparticles at 20 and 40 mg/kg showed abnormal structures of the cell, as well as nanoparticle deposition in the cytoplasm and nuclear membrane of tested orangs at 40 mg/kg concentration.

Doudi and Setorki [61] treated the experimental rats with different concentrations of copper nanoparticles (10, 100, and 300 mg/kg) after they studied the effects on the liver and lungs. The results of their work have been shown to cause structural changes in cells of the liver and lungs at high doses. Another work by Lei et al. [62] took tissue sections from the liver and kidney of rats that were treated with 100 and 200 mg/kg of copper nanoparticles once a day for 5 days. The necrosis in the liver has been noted at 200 mg/kg with structural changes in the kidney, while there was no alteration in the structure of the liver and kidney cells at 100 mg/kg. Wang et al. [63] studied the effects of various concentrations of copper nanoparticles on rats. Their study explored histological alterations in the liver, spleen, and kidney in male and female rats at 1250 and 2500 mg/kg.

The previous studies of the effects of silver and copper nanoparticles on the organs of rats at various doses of nanoparticles above concluded that the high doses showed clear accumulation and toxic effects of nanoparticles *in vivo* studies. While at low doses, there were no histological changes in the rats with safe use. Future work is required to clarify the biological effects of silver and copper nanoparticles using animal models.

5. Conclusions

The pathogenicity of Staphylococcal, especially *Staphylococcus aureus*, is widespread in nosocomial infections and long hospitality treatment periods between patients. However, *Staphylococcus epidermidis* has a recent history of pathogenicity with inflammation wounds. The drugs used in the protocol of treatment for bacterial infection are antibiotics. Widespread use of antibiotics produces problems for medical scientists related to resistant bacteria to these drugs. These problems come from transport genes responsible for resistance from honor plasmid to receiving plasmid in bacteria.

The development of a new generation of antibiotics takes time and is expansive at the same time. Using a new drug with excellent bactericide activity is a recent option to solve this problem in the medicine sector. Nanoscience is one of the options selected to solve this challenge. A number of inorganic nanoparticles have been synthesized using biological methods. Silver nanoparticles have been approved for their activity against many pathogens, including *S. aureus* and *S. epidermidis*, depending on several scientific reviews without resistance bacteria to it. The other inorganic nanoparticles, such as copper nanoparticles, have been reviewed, and the activity of copper nanoparticles toward several human pathogens of *S. aureus* and a limited number of *S. epidermidis* has been reviewed.

Antibiotics have a known mechanism of activity against bacteria. In comparison with silver and copper nanoparticles, they have antibacterial activity but no clear mechanism, such as in antibiotics. Four suggested hypotheses about the mechanism of inorganic silver and copper nanoparticles have been discussed. The nanoparticles first adhere and accumulate on the cell walls of bacteria. The second hypothesis suggested transporting the nanoparticles of silver and copper passed through the pore in the cell wall and reached the surface of the cell membrane. Some of the nanoparticles that accumulated on the surface of the cell membrane worked to modify the permeability of the cell membrane and disturb the respiration process in the cell membrane of bacteria, resulting in the entry of harmful materials inside the cell, causing death to bacteria. The nanoparticles that successfully passed the cell membrane using channel of ion exchange or proteins channel or even through the self-membrane of cell because they have tiny small size compared with the size of the membrane reacted with the DNA molecules causing an inhibition of the DNA replication, and because of that, there is no transcription and translation happened. The last hypothesis talked about the creation of reactive oxygen radicals. This product is considered toxic to cells. More investigated studies *in vivo* as animal models need to study the safety of the nanoparticles to use them as drugs.

Conflict of interest

The authors declare no conflict of interest.

Author details

Abdalmohaimen Suood[1*], Iman Mahdi[2] and Mahmood Saleh[2]

1 Directorate of Salah al-Din Education, Ministry of Education, Ishaqi, Iraq

2 University of Tikrit, Tikrit, Iraq

*Address all correspondence to: mohaimen@st.tu.edu.iq

References

[1] Chessa D, Ganau G, Mazzarello V. An overview of *Staphylococcus epidermidis* and *Staphylococcus aureus* with a focus on developing countries. The Journal of Infection in Developing Countries. 2015;**9**:547-550. DOI: 10.3855/jidc.6923

[2] Oliver LV, Calduch PB, Rodríguez LF, Ortega DN, Samper AMD, Rodríguez JC. Methicillin-resistant *Staphylococcus epidermidis* infectious keratitis: Clinical and microbiological profile. Revista Española de Quimioterapia. 2022;**35**:171-177. DOI: 10.37201/req/128.2021

[3] Ahmed AA, Hamzah H, Maaroof M. Analyzing formation of silver nanoparticles from the filamentous fungus *Fusarium oxysporum* and their antimicrobial activity. Turkish Journal of Biology. 2018;**42**:54-62. DOI: 10.3906/biy-1710-2

[4] Suood AM, Saleh MK, Thalij KM. The inhibition ability of copper nanoparticles synthesized by green tea extract on healing the induced contaminated wounds in laboratory hamsters. Materials Today: Proceedings. 2022;**61**:774-780. DOI: 10. 1016/j.matpr.2021.09.035

[5] Lowy FD. *Staphylococcus aureus* infections. New England Journal of Medicine. 1998;**339**:520-532. DOI: 10.1056/NEJM199808203390806

[6] Otto M. *Staphylococcus epidermidis*—the' accidental' pathogen. Nature Reviews Microbiology. 2009;**7**:555-567. DOI: doi.org/10.1038/nrmicro2182

[7] Rogers KL, Fey PD, Rupp ME. Coagulase-negative staphylococcal infections. Infectious Disease Clinics of North America. 2009;**23**:73-98. DOI: doi.org/10.1016/j.idc.2008.10.001

[8] De Beer J, Brysiewicz P, Bhengu BR. Intensive care nursing in South Africa. Southern African Journal of Critical Care. 2011;**27**:6-10

[9] Vuong C, Otto M. *Staphylococcus epidermidis* infections. Microbes and Infection. 2002;**4**:481-489. DOI: 10.1016/S1286-4579(02)01563-0

[10] Frígols B, Martí M, Salesa B, Hernández-Oliver C, Aarstad O, Teialeret Ulset AS, et al. Graphene oxide in zinc alginate films: Antibacterial activity, cytotoxicity, zinc release, water sorption/diffusion, wettability and opacity. PLoS One. 2019;**2019**(14):e0212819. DOI: 10.1371/journal.pone.0212819

[11] Hulla JE, Sahu SC, Hayes AW. Nanotechnology: History and future. Human & Experimental Toxicology. 2015;**34**(12):1318-1321. DOI: 10.1177/096032711560 3588

[12] Hossen S, Hossain MK, Basher MK, Mia MNH, Rahman MT, Uddin MJ. Smart nanocarrier-based drug delivery systems for cancer therapy and toxicity studies: A review. Journal of Advanced Research. 2019;**15**:1-18. DOI: 10.1016/j.jare.2018. 06.005

[13] Spirescu VA, Chircov C, Grumezescu AM, Vasile BȘ, Andronescu E. Inorganic nanoparticles and composite films for antimicrobial therapies. International Journal of Molecular Sciences. 2021;**22**:4595. DOI: 10.3390/ijms22094595

[14] Bhardwaj AK, Naraian R. Cyanobacteria as biochemical energy source for the synthesis of inorganic nanoparticles, mechanism and potential applications. A Review.

3 Biotech. 2021;**11**:1-16. DOI: 10.1007/s13205-021-02992-5

[15] Dash KK, Deka P, Bangar SP, Chaudhary V, Trif M, Rusu A. Applications of inorganic nanoparticles in food packaging: A comprehensive review. Polymers. 2022;**14**:521. DOI: 10.3390/polym14030521

[16] Zhang XF, Liu ZG, Shen W, Gurunathan S. Silver nanoparticles: Synthesis, characterization, properties, applications, and therapeutic approaches. International Journal of Molecular Sciences. 2016;**17**:1534. DOI: 10.3390/ijms17091534

[17] Yaqoob AA, Umar K, Ibrahim MNM. Silver nanoparticles: various methods of synthesis, size affecting factors and their potential applications–A review. Applied Nanoscience. 2020;**10**:1369-1378. DOI: 10.1007/s13204-020-01318-w

[18] AbdelRahim K, Mahmoud SY, Ali AM, Almaary KS, Mustafa AEZM, Husseiny SM. Extracellular biosynthesis of silver nanoparticles using *Rhizopus stolonifer*. Saudi Journal of Biological Sciences. 2017;**24**:208-216. DOI: 10.1016/j.sjbs.2016.02.025

[19] Sadowski Z, Maliszewska IH, Grochowalska B, Polowczyk I, Kozlecki T. Synthesis of silver nanoparticles using microorganisms. Materials Science-Poland. 2008;**26**:419-424

[20] Ahmed S, Ahmad M, Swami BL, Ikram S. A review on plants extract mediated synthesis of silver nanoparticles for antimicrobial applications: a green expertise. Journal of Advanced Research. 2016;**7**:17-28. DOI: 10.1016/j.jare.2015.02.007

[21] Marin S, Mihail Vlasceanu G, Elena Tiplea R, Raluca Bucur I, Lemnaru M, Minodora Marin M, et al. Applications and toxicity of silver nanoparticles: A recent review. Current Topics in Medicinal Chemistry. 2015;**15**:1596-1604

[22] Pubmed.ncbi.nlm.nih.gov web site. Activity. silver nanoparticles. Pathogen. *Staphylococcus aureus* 2022. Available from: https://pubmed.ncbi.nlm.nih.gov/?term=Activity.+silver+nanoparticles.+Pathogen.+Staphylococcus+aureus&filter=simsearch1.fha&filter=journalcategory.medline [Accessed: August 27, 2022]

[23] Shahverdi RA, Fakhimi A, Shahverdi HR, Minaian S. Synthesis and effect of silver nanoparticles on the antibacterial activity of different antibiotics against *Staphyloccocus aureus* and *Escherichia coli*. Nanomedicine: Nanotechnology, Biology and Medicine. 2007;**3**:168-171. DOI: 10.1016/j.nano.2007.02.001

[24] Wan G, Ruan L, Yin Y, Yang T, Ge M, Cheng X. Effects of silver nanoparticles in combination with antibiotics on the resistant bacteria *Acinetobacter baumannii*. International Journal of Nanomedicine. 2016;**2016**(11):3789-3800. DOI: 10.2147/IJN.S104166

[25] Xu N, Cheng H, Xu J, Li F, Gao B, Li Z, et al. Silver-loaded nanotubular structures enhanced bactericidal efficiency of antibiotics with synergistic effect *in vitro* and *in vivo*. International Journal of Nanomedicine. 2017;**12**:731-743. DOI: 10.2147/IJN.S123648

[26] Elbehiry A, Al-Dubaib M, Marzouk E, Moussa I. Antibacterial effects and resistance induction of silver and gold nanoparticles against *Staphylococcus aureus*-induced mastitis and the potential toxicity in rats. Microbiology. 2019;**8**:e00698. DOI: 10.1002/mbo3.698

[27] Panáček A, Kvítek L, Smékalová M, Večeřová R, Kolář M,

Röderová M, et al. Bacterial resistance to silver nanoparticles and how to overcome it. Nature Nanotechnology. 2018;**13**:65-71. DOI: 10.1038/s41565-017-0013-y

[28] Chakraborty R, Basu T. Metallic copper nanoparticles induce apoptosis in a human skin melanoma A-375 cell line. Nanotechnology. 2017;**28**:105101. DOI: 10.1088/1361-6528/aa57b0

[29] Esteban-Cubillo A, Pecharromán C, Aguilar E, Santarén J, Moya JS. Antibacterial activity of copper monodispersed nanoparticles into sepiolite. Journal of Materials Science. 2006;**2006**(41):5208-5212. DOI: 10.1007/s10853-006-0432-x

[30] Ranjitham AM, Ranjani GS, Caroling G. Biosynthesis, characterization, antimicrobial activity of copper nanoparticles using fresh aqueous *Ananas comosus* L.(Pineapple) extract. International Journal of PharmTech Research. 2015;**8**:750-769

[31] Nasrollahzadeh M, Sajadi SM. Green synthesis of copper nanoparticles using *Ginkgo biloba* L. leaf extract and their catalytic activity for the Huisgen [3+ 2] cycloaddition of azides and alkynes at room temperature. Journal of Colloid and Interface Science. 2015, 2015;**457**:141-147. DOI: 10.1016/j.jcis.2015.07.004

[32] Kalpana VN, Chakraborthy P, Palanichamy V, Rajeswari VD. Synthesis and characterization of copper nanoparticles using Tridax procumbens and its application in degradation of bismarck brown. Analysis. 2016;**2016**(9):498-507

[33] Khodashenas B, Ghorbani HR. Synthesis of copper nanoparticles: An overview of the various methods. Korean Journal of Chemical Engineering. 2014;**31**:1105-1109. DOI: 10.1007/s11814-014-0127-y

[34] Patel BH, Channiwala MZ, Chaudhari SB, Mandot AA. Biosynthesis of copper nanoparticles; its characterization and efficacy against human pathogenic bacterium. Journal of Environmental Chemical Engineering. 2016;**4**:2163-2169. DOI: 10.1016/j.jece.2016.03.046

[35] Din MI, Rehan R. Synthesis, characterization, and applications of copper nanoparticles. Analytical Letters. 2017;**50**:50-62. DOI: 10.1080/00032719.20 16.1172081

[36] Wong-Pinto LS, Mercado A, Chong G, Salazar P, Ordóñez JI. Biosynthesis of copper nanoparticles from copper tailings ore–An approach to the 'Bionanomining'. Journal of Cleaner Production. 2021;**315**:128107. DOI: 10.1016/j.jclepro.2021. 128107

[37] Usman MS, El Zowalaty ME, Shameli K, Zainuddin N, Salama M, Ibrahim NA. Synthesis, characterization, and antimicrobial properties of copper nanoparticles. International Journal of Nanomedicine. 2013;**8**:4467-4479. DOI: 10.2147/IJN.S50837

[38] Yoon KY, Byeon JH, Park JH, Hwang J. Susceptibility constants of *Escherichia coli* and *Bacillus subtilis* to silver and copper nanoparticles. Science of the Total Environment. 2007;**373**:572-575. DOI: 10.1016/j.scitotenv.2006.11.007

[39] Pubmed.ncbi.nlm.nih.gov web site. copper nanoparticles against *Staphylococcus aureus*. 2022. Available from: https://pubmed.ncbi.nlm.nih.gov/?term=copper+nanoparticles+against+Staphylococcus+aureus.&filter=simsearch1.fha&filter=journalcategory.medline. [Accessed: August 27, 2022]

[40] Suood AM, Saleh MK, Thalij KM. Synthesis of copper nanoparticles using aspergillus niger and their efficacy

against pathogenic *Staphylococcus aureus*. In: IOP Conference Series: Earth and Environmental Science. Vol. 910. Babil, Iraq: Fourth International Conference for Agricultural and Sustainability Sciences; 2021. p. 012083. DOI: 10.1088/1755-1315/910/1/012083

[41] Abbasi A, Ghorban K, Nojoomi F, Dadmanesh M. Smaller copper oxide nanoparticles have more biological effects versus breast cancer and nosocomial infections bacteria. The Asian Pacific Journal of Cancer Prevention. 2021;**22**:893-902. DOI: 10.31557/APJ CP.2021.22.3.893

[42] Kruk T, Szczepanowicz K, Stefańska J, Socha RP, Warszyński P. Synthesis and antimicrobial activity of monodisperse copper nanoparticles. Colloids and Surfaces B: Biointerfaces. 2015;**128**:17-22. DOI: 10.1016/j.colsurfb.2015.02.009

[43] Selvarani M. Investigation of the synergistic antibacterial action of copper nanoparticles on certain antibiotics against human pathogens. International Journal of Pharmacy and Pharmaceutical Sciences. 2018;**10**:83-86. DOI: 10.22159/ijpps.2018 v10i 10.28069

[44] Woźniak-Budych MJ, Przysiecka Ł, Langer K, Peplińska B, Jarek M, Wiesner M, et al. Green synthesis of rifampicin-loaded copper nanoparticles with enhanced antimicrobial activity. Journal of Materials Science: Materials in Medicine. 2017;**28**:1-16. DOI: 10.1007/s10856-017-5857-z

[45] Willey JM, Sherwood L, Woolverton CJ. Prescott's Microbiology. 9 th ed. New York: McGraw-Hill; 2014. p. 189

[46] Durán N, Marcato PD, Conti RD, Alves OL, Costa F, Brocchi M. Potential use of silver nanoparticles on pathogenic bacteria, their toxicity and possible mechanisms of action. Journal of the Brazilian Chemical Society. 2010;**21**:949-959. DOI: 10.1590/S0103-50532010000600002

[47] Durán N, Durán M, De Jesus MB, Seabra AB, Fávaro WJ, Nakazato G. Silver nanoparticles: A new view on mechanistic aspects on antimicrobial activity. Nanomedicine: Nanotechnology, Biology and Medicine. 2016;**12**:789-799. DOI: 10. 1016/j.nano.2015.11.016

[48] Tang S, Zheng J. Antibacterial activity of silver nanoparticles: Structural effects. Advanced Healthcare Materials. 2018;**7**:1701503. DOI: 10.1002/adhm.201701 503

[49] Tran QH, Le AT. Silver nanoparticles: Synthesis, properties, toxicology, applications and perspectives. Advances in natural sciences. Nanoscience and Nanotechnology. 2013;**4**:033001. DOI: 2043-6254/18/049501+2$33.00

[50] Sondi I, Salopek-Sondi B. Silver nanoparticles as antimicrobial agent: A case study on *E. coli* as a model for Gram-negative bacteria. Journal of Colloid and Interface Science. 2004;**275**:177-182. DOI: 10.1016/j.jcis.2004.02.012

[51] Gogoi SK, Gopinath P, Paul A, Ramesh A, Ghosh SS, Chattopadhyay A. Green fluorescent protein-expressing *Escherichia coli* as a model system for investigating the antimicrobial activities of silver nanoparticles. Langmuir. 2006;**22**:9322-9328. DOI: 10.1021/la060661v

[52] Morones JR, Elechiguerra JL, Camacho A, Holt K, Kouri JB, Ramírez JT, et al. The bactericidal effect of silver nanoparticles. Nanotechnology. 2005;**16**:2346-2353. DOI: 10.1088/0957-4484/16/10/059

[53] Ruparelia JP, Chatterjee AK, Duttagupta SP, Mukherji S. Strain specificity in antimicrobial activity of silver and copper nanoparticles. Acta Biomaterialia. 2008;**4**:707-716. DOI: 10.1016/j.actbio.2007.11.006

[54] Schrand AM, Rahman MF, Hussain SM, Schlager JJ, Smith DA, Syed AF. Metal-based nanoparticles and their toxicity assessment. WIREs Nanomedicine and Nanobiotechnology. 2010;**2**:554-568. DOI: 10.1002/wnan.103

[55] Ren G, Hu D, Cheng EW, Vargas-Reus MA, Reip P, Allaker RP. Characterization of copper oxide nanoparticles for antimicrobial applications. International Journal of Antimicrobial Agents. 2009;**33**:587-590. DOI: 10.1016/j.ijantimicag.2008.12.00 4

[56] Kim J, Cho H, Ryu S, Choi M. Effects of metal ions on the activity of protein tyrosine phosphatase VHR: Highly potent and reversible oxidative inactivation by Cu2+ ion. Archives of Biochemistry and Biophysics. 2000;**382**:72-80. DOI: 10.1006/abbi. 2000.1996

[57] Deryabin DG, Aleshina ES, Vasilchenko AS, Deryabina TD, Efremova LV, Karimov IF, et al. Investigation of copper nanoparticles antibacterial mechanisms tested by luminescent *Escherichia coli* strains. Nanotechnologies in Russia. 2013;*8*:402-408. DOI: 10.1134/S19950780130300 63

[58] Nakkala JR, Mata R, Raja K, Khub Chandra V, Sadras SR. Green synthesized silver nanoparticles: Catalytic dye degradation, *in vitro* anticancer activity and *in vivo* toxicity in rats. Materials Science and Engineering C. 2018;**1**(91):372-381. DOI: 10.1016/j.msec.2018.05.048

[59] Kim WY, Kim J, Park JD, Ryu HY, Yu IJ. Histological study of gender differences in accumulation of silver nanoparticles in kidneys of Fischer 344 rats. Journal of Toxicology and Environmental Health. 2009;**72**:1279-1284. DOI: 10.1080/1528739090 3212287

[60] Tiwari DK, Jin T, Behari J. Dose-dependent in-vivo toxicity assessment of silver nanoparticle in Wistar rats. Toxicology Mechanisms and Methods. 2011 Jan;**21**:13-24. DOI: 10.3109/15376516.2010.529184

[61] Doudi M, Setorki M. Acute effect of nano-copper on liver tissue and function in rat. Nanomedicine Journal. 2014;**1**:331-338

[62] Lei R, Yang B, Wu C, Liao M, Ding R, Wang Q. Mitochondrial dysfunction and oxidative damage in the liver and kidney of rats following exposure to copper nanoparticles for five consecutive days. Toxicology Research. 2015;**4**:351-364. DOI: 10.1039/c4tx00156g

[63] Wang D, Lin Z, Wang T, Yao Z, Qin M, Zheng S, et al. Where does the toxicity of metal oxide nanoparticles come from: The nanoparticles, the ions, or a combination of both. Journal of Hazardous Materials. 2016;**5**(308):328-334. DOI: 10.1016/j.jhazmat. 2016.01.066

Chapter 8

Potential Use of African Botanicals and Other Compounds in the Treatment of Methicillin-Resistant *Staphylococcus aureus* Infections

Enitan Omobolanle Adesanya
and Akingbolabo Daniel Ogunlakin

Abstract

Infections caused by the group of *Staphylococcus* bacteria are commonly called Staph infections, and over 30 types of Staphylococcal bacteria exist with *Staphylococcus aureus* causing about 90% of the infections from the genus. *Staphylococcus aureus* (*S. aureus*) is a major cause of both hospital- and community-acquired infections with major concern arising from its strain of species that is resistant to many antibiotics. One of such strain is the Methicillin-resistant *Staphylococcus aureus* (MRSA) that has been described to be a resistance to methicillin drugs. Another is glycopeptides-resistant emerging from the increased use of glycopeptides drugs. This continuous emergence and spread of new resistant strains of *S. aureus* is a major challenge which makes the search for novel anti-resistant agents imperative. The development of vaccines from natural and synthetic products is some of the measures being proposed for the protection against the infections. Also, the development of monoclonal or polyclonal antibodies for passive immunization is sought for, and attentions with regard to arriving at successful trials have been directed back to medicinal plant research as an alternative. This review discusses the treatment strategies of MRSA, the antibacterial property of various medicinal plants, and the influence of their active compounds on methicillin-resistant *S. aureus* (MRSA), as well as to recommend the path to future research in this area.

Keywords: staphylococcal infections, vaccines, medicinal plants

1. Introduction

Staphylococcus is a genus in the Bacillales order that belongs to the Staphylococcaceae family. Microscopically, they appear spherical and form grape-like clusters. The genus is a Gram-positive bacterium, and their species are facultative anaerobic organisms, meaning they can grow in both aerobic and anaerobic environments. The genus contains approximately 30 species, nine of which have two subspecies, including one three subspecies and the other with four subspecies [1].

IntechOpen

Many species in the genus do not cause disease and typically live just on skin and mucous membranes of animals and humans. *Staphylococcus* species have been identified as nectar-inhabiting microbes and a minor component of the soil microbiome [2]. Among the bacteria in this genus, five are considered potential human pathogens: *S. aureus*, *S. epidermidis*, *S. saprophiticus*, *S. haemolyticus*, and *S. hominis*, with the first three species the most common. However, *S.aureus* is considered as the most dangerous pathogen, and one of the *Staphylococcus* species is capable of coagulating plasma [3].

2. Types of staphylococcal infections

There are numerous types of infections caused by *Staphylococcus* bacteria, which are frequently found on the skin or in the nose of many healthy people. These infections are usually harmless or can cause minor skin infections [2]. However, infections can be fatal when bacteria enter the bloodstream, joints, bones, lungs, or heart and are thus regarded to as bloodstream pathogenic bacteria [4]. As a result, a number of otherwise healthy people are developing potentially fatal staphylococcal infections [5]. Although these infections are communicable and can be acquired by sneezing, coughing, or touching an infected wound, many cases occur when an individual comes into contact with contaminated items such as a wet towel, remote control, or door handle. Similarly, direct personal encounter with an infected person can allow the spread of the infection [4]. There have been several staphylococcal infections ranging from skin infections that cause open sores to bloodstream infections widely recognized as bacteremia infestation of the bone to endocarditis, septicaemia an infectious disease of the heart lining, food poisoning, pneumonia, and toxic shock syndrome (TSS) (a life-threatening predicament caused by contaminants from certain kinds of bacteria) [6].

3. Risk factors for staphylococcal infections

Since *Staphylococcus* bacteria are commensal organisms, anyone can develop a staphylococcal infection. However, some people are at higher risk, including those who have a chronic medical condition including hyperglycemia, cancer, vascular disease, eczema, and lung disease, a compromised immune system such as HIV/AIDS, on medications to prevent organ rejection, or chemotherapy. Likewise, those who have recently had surgery and those who use a catheter, breathing tube, or feeding through tube are susceptible to Staph infection [7]. Those on dialysis and those who use illegal drugs to participate in contact sports are also at high risk [8]. For the latter, the drugs increase the rate of sweating; thus, it encourages skin-to-skin interaction with other people or via device sharing.

3.1 Drug resistance

When an infection occurs, antibiotics are prescribed for treatment based on the type of infection. Such treatments can come in the form of a lotion, ointment, medications (to swallow), or intravenous (IV) injection, while surgery is proposed for bone infectious diseases [4]. Although antibiotics are used, there have been cases where it does not work; hence, we say that the *Staphylococcus* bacterium has grown resistant to the antibiotics. The different species of *Staphylococcus* have cases of antibiotic resistance, but widespread prevalence of antibiotic resistance strains are commonly found in the *Staphylococcus aureus* known as methicillin-resistant *Staphylococcus aureus* (MRSA) [9].

Staphylococcus aureus has now been confirmed to be resistant to many antimicrobial agents over the last few decades, but it has recently become tolerant to daptomycin and linezolid, two of the most recent lines of therapies [10]. *Staphylococcus aureus* bacteria is a member of the ESKAPE pathogens comprising of *Enterococcus faecium*, *S. aureus*, *Klebsiella spp.*, *Acinetobacter baumannii*, *Pseudomonas aeruginosa,* and *Enterobacter spp.*, which are capable of "escaping" the biocidal action of antibiotics and jointly representing new paradigms in pathogenesis, transmission, and resistance group of bacteria, all of which have multidrug resistance profiles [11]. Although MRSA infections have decreased in the United States, Europe, Canada, and South Africa, an increase has been observed in some regions, including sub-Saharan Africa, raising public health concerns [12].

3.2 Mechanisms and site of resistance

There are several antibacterial resistance molecular mechanisms. One example is intrinsic antibacterial resistance, which can be found in the genetic composition of bacterial strains. For example, an antibiotic target may be missing from the bacterial genome but acquired resistance from a chromosomal mutation or the acquirement of extra-chromosomal DNA [13]. Furthermore, antibacterial-producing bacteria have developed defense mechanisms that have been found to be similar to antibacterial-resistant strains and may have been transferred to them. Furthermore, antibacterial resistance is frequently spread via vertical transmission of gene mutation during growth and genetic recombination of DNA via horizontal genetic transfer [14]. Antibacterial resistance genes, for example, can be interchanged among various bacterial strains or species through plasmids carrying these resistant gene [15]. Plasmids containing multiple resistance genes can bestow resistance to various antibacterial agents [15]. Also, cross-resistance to the many antibacterial could indeed arise if a resistance mechanism encrypted by a specific gene expresses resistance to even more than one antibacterial chemical agent [15, 16].

Antibacterial-resistant species, dubbed "superbugs," are now contributing to the onset of diseases that were previously under control. Newly emerging bacterial strains usually cause tuberculosis which are tolerant to subsequently good antimicrobial therapies, for example, pose numerous therapeutic challenges, as does New Delhi metallo-β-lactamase-1 (NDM-1), a newly identified enzyme that transmits bacterial resistance to a wide spectrum of beta-lactam antibacterial agents [17]. According to a report published by the United Kingdom's Health Protection Agency, "thus many isolates with NDM-1 enzyme are tolerant to all conventional intravenous antibiotics prescribed to treat severe infections" [18].

3.3 The management of staphylococcal infections

Regardless of the fact that several novel antimicrobial drugs have just been developed, resistance rate to them has managed to increase and has become serious challenge as we run out of candidates' drug. Antimicrobial resistance issues are being addressed both in healthcare and community configurations, necessitating a multidisciplinary approach involving many different collaborators across the care continuum. For instance, in a survey report by Okwu et al. [19], 18–33 percent of the total *S. aureus*-infected patients went on to develop MRSA infections. Community-acquired methicillin-resistant *Staphylococcus aureus* strains (CA-MRSA) are also becoming more common in hospital-onset MRSA infections. As stated by the Centers for Disease Control and Prevention (CDC), antibiotic resistance causes more than 2 million ailments and 23,000 deaths in the United States each year [20].

Methicillin-resistant *Staphylococcus aureus* has gained worldwide popularity, and its incidence has risen in both care services and community-based settings. MRSA prevalence varied by country, for example, 0.4% through Sweden [21]; 25% in Western India to 50% through Southern India [22]; 33%–43% in Nigeria [19]; and 37–56% in Greece, Portugal, and Romania in 2014 [23]. Also, MRSA has been found in hospitals all over the world, with rates exceeding 50% in Asia, Malta, North and South America, and Europe [24, 25]. Its prevalence rates varied due to various prevalence factors including geographic location and health service capacity to run infection control programs [26]. Akanbi and Mbe [27] found vancomycin-resistant *Staphylococcus aureus* (VRSA) in clinical isolates ranging from 0% to 6% in southern Nigeria, and 57.7% across Zaria, the northern part of Nigeria.

Likewise, vancomycin resistance was found in 1.4% of *S. aureus* isolates through Southern India [28]. Other countries, including Australia, Korea, Hong Kong, Scotland, Israel, Thailand, and South Africa, have reported *S. aureus* with reduced vancomycin sensitivity, with prevalence ranging from 0 to 74% [29–31]. Despite the frequent use of vancomycin in the treatment of pathogens, numerous researchers have documented vancomycin intermediate *Staphylococcus aureus* (VISA) and vancomycin-resistant *Staphylococcus aureus* (VRSA) occurrences [32–34]. Teicoplanin, daptomycin, linezolid, and other costly drugs are currently used to treat bacteria with low vancomycin sensitivity. However, global resistance to these drugs has been identified [22, 35–38]. The MRSA infection remains a significant issue all over the globe and also a therapeutic challenge due to the scarcity and high cost of antibacterial agents. The increasing existence of MRSA infections, changing antibiotic resistance, and involvement in hospital and community infections have an influence on the use and treatment outcomes of previously existing anti-infective compounds [39].

Plants have been used for centuries to treat illnesses and diseases. Plant extracts are being studied as medicines, because several studies have shown that their crude extracts possess antimicrobial effect and could be excellent substitutes for current antibiotics. Recent published reports suggest that medicinal plants with anti-MRSA activity may be taken into account as medication of MRSA infections [36, 40].

3.4 Medicinal plants and staphylococcal infections

Natural products, such as medicinal herbs, have contributed significantly to human wellbeing and drug development. Ethno-medicinal plants have the possibility to be effective therapeutically. Over 80% of patients in many developing countries, including Nigeria, treat contagious diseases with home-made herbal remedies. Regardless of whether Western medicine is available in certain localities, medicinal plants are still extensively utilized because of their effectiveness, relevance, and low cost. Although all parts of the plant are utilized in traditional therapies and can therefore act as lead compounds, they are also promising sources of novel pharmaceutical substances. Recent years have seen a substantial growth in the utilization of natural remedies for human wellbeing and as blueprints for developing newer beneficial pharmaceuticals around the world [41].

The emergence of multidrug-resistant pathogenic organisms associated with the overuse and misuse of antibacterial agents has compelled the World Health Organization (WHO) to acknowledge and make known the pressing need to find unique antibiotic and/or innovative techniques to combat the global threat posed by them [42]. This has resulted in a resurgence of research in traditional medicines [43]. **Table 1** shows the various mechanisms of medicinal plants and their bioactive compounds. Their mechanisms of action includes increased cell wall membrane penetrability, downregulation of efflux pump systems, reconfiguration of the active site or enzymatic ruin, and modification of bacterial enzymes [61].

Several studies have demonstrated that several phytoconstituents possess antibacterial effect against MRSA. On the tested MRSA strains, the plants' minimum inhibitory levels (MICs) varied widely from 1.25 g/mL to 6.30 mg/mL. Some medicinal herbs had minimum inhibitory concentration of 1.0 mg/mL, whereas few herbs had MIC values that were higher than 1.0 mg/mL and much less than 8.0 mg/mL. Extracts with minimum inhibitory concentration less than 8 mg/mL are broadly acknowledged to have antibacterial effects, whereas those with values less than 1 mg/mL have been classified as exceptional [41, 62].

3.5 Plants' secondary metabolites and treatment of staphylococcal infection

Botanicals are good source of different classes of phytochemicals. Plants produce phytoconstituents, also referred to as secondary metabolites, as natural biological agents in response to external and abiotic stresses. They are essential for the survival and defense of plants. Polyphenols, alkaloids, steroids, essential oils, saponins, as well as other compounds are among them. They possess antimutagenic, antitumor, free radical scavenging, antiseptic, and anti-inflammatory properties, which contribute to plants' pharmacological potency [63].

Ethanol and methanol have been the most commonly used solvents for isolation and purification of anti-MRSA molecules from medicinal herbs. This is because alcoholic extracts have a stronger antibacterial property than aqueous extracts. Ethanolic extracts had already been discovered to have stronger antimicrobial properties than aqueous extracts due to the existence of more polyphenols. Ethanol is more effective at breaking down cell membranes and seeds, enabling polyphenols to be released from cells. Another enzyme, polyphenol oxidase, which degrades polyphenols in aqueous extracts, is rendered ineffective in both methanol and ethanol. Additionally, water is an excellent medium for the growth of microorganisms than alcohol [64].

Despite being more ionic than ethanol, methanol is not commonly used in plant extraction because of its cytotoxic nature, which might lead to false-positive findings [65]. The pharmacological influences of these botanicals and their constituents could be utilized in drug development [63]. The phytochemicals in these plants are responsible for their antibacterial (including anti-MRSA) activity through several mechanisms. For example, flavonoids form complex ions with bacterial cell membrane, extracellular proteins, and soluble proteins, meanwhile tannins restrict microbial adhesions, enzymes, as well as cell encircling proteins (**Table 1**) [58, 66–69].

3.6 African medicinal plants' efficacy against staphylococcal infections

Six Nigerian medicinal plants, Bambara (*Terminalia avicennioides*), *Bushveld peacock-berry* (*Phylantus discoideus*), Bridelia (*Bridella ferruginea*), billygoat-weed (*Ageratum conyzoides*), basil (*Ocimum gratissimum*), and *copperleaf* (*Acalypha*

Plant	Part/solvent for extraction	Dose (MIC)	Active constituents	Mode of action	Reference
Allium sativum	Rhizhome			Inhibition of cell wall synthesis; Inhibition of cell membrane function	[44]
Pimenta dioica	Essential oil			Inhibition of MRSA growth	[45]
Aloe vera	Leaf exudate			inhibition of protein synthesis	[44]
Alpinia galangal	Rhizhome			Inhibition of cell wall synthesis; Inhibition of cell membrane function	[44]
Cinnamomum camphora	Essential oil		Camphor	Inhibiting MRSA growth	[45]
Canarium odontophyllum	Leaves/ methanol Leaves/acetone	312.5 μg/mL 156.25 μg/m	Saponin	Bactericidal action	[46]
Cinnamomum zeylanicum	Essential oil			Inhibition of MRSA growth	[45]
Salvia sclarea	Essential oil			Inhibition of MRSA growth	[45]
Syzygium aromaticum	Essential oil			Inhibition of MRSA growth	[45]
Curcuma domestica	Rhizhome			Inhibition of cell membrane function; inhibition of protein synthesis	[44]
Curcuma xanthorrhiza	Rhizhome			Inhibition of cell membrane function	[44]
Citrus paradise	Essential oil			Inhibition of MRSA growth	[45]
Cymbopogon citratus	Essential oil			Inhibition of MRSA growth	[45]
Lippa citriodora	Essential oil	55 μl/ml		Cytotoxicity	[47]
Phoenix dactylifera	Seed/ Nanoparticles of aqueous extract	0.67 ± 0.94 μg/ml		Electrostatic attraction between positively charged AgNPs and negatively charged teichoic acid in MRSA cell membrane results in an increase in membrane fluidity and, eventually, destabilization and depletion of intracellular components.	[48]

Plant	Part/solvent for extraction	Dose (MIC)	Active constituents	Mode of action	Reference
Piper bettle	Leaves			Inhibition of cell membrane function	[44]
Plectranthus amboinicus	Leaves/ hydroalcoholic extract	18.7–9.3 mg/mL	Carvacrol	Modification of the constitution to increase the fluidity of the cell membrane	[49–51]
Quercus infectoria	Galls/methanol	0.625 mg/mL		Post-antibiotic effect; destruction of bacterial cell wall.	[52]
	Galls/acetone	0.3125 mg/mL			
Rhazya stricta	Leaves/aqueous			Bactericidal action	[53]
Sambucus nigra	Flower or berry/water		Tannins (derivatives of gallic acid, hydroxycinnamic acid, caffeic acid) and terpenes		[54]
Syzygium polyanthum	Leaves			Inhibition of cell membrane function; inhibition of cell wall synthesis	[44]
Thymus vulgaris	Essential oil			Inhibition of MRSA growth	[45]
Gaultheria procumbens	Essential oil			Inhibition of MRSA growth	[45]
Zingiber officinale	Rhizhome			Inhibition of cell membrane function	[44]
Eleutherine Americana	Bulb	0.78 µg/mL	Eleucanainones A	Downregulation of basal expression of agrA, cidA, icaA, and sarA in methicillin-resistant S. aureus	[55]
		3.12 µg/mL	Eleucanainones B	Bactericidal action	
Anethum graveolens	Essential oil		α-phellandrene, *p*-cymene and carvone	Topical administration on the MRSA-infected wound in BALB/c male mice significantly elevates Bcl-2 expression which then triggers cellular proliferation.	[56]
Boswellia papyrifera	Oleo-gum resin/methanol	62.5 to 500 µg/ml		Bactericidal action	[57]
Commiphora molmol	oleo-gum resin/methanol	31.25 and 250 µg/m		Bactericidal action	[57]
Garcinia mangostana	Ethanol	0.05–0.4 mg/ mL		Bactericidal action	[58]
Punica granatum	Ethanol	0.2–0.4 mg/mL		Bactericidal action	[58]

Plant	Part/solvent for extraction	Dose (MIC)	Active constituents	Mode of action	Reference
Quercus infectori	Ethanol	0.2–0.4 mg/mL		Bactericidal action	[58]
Glycyrrhiza glabra	Rhizomes/ethanol	50–100 μg/mL	Isoliquiritigenin	Drug resistance reversal effect	[59]
			Liquiritigenin	Drug resistance reversal effect	
Cordia latifolia	Methanol			Anti-MRSA effect	[60]
Thymus vulgaris	Methanol			Anti-MRSA effect	[60]

Table 1.
Mechanisms of medicinal plants against MRSA bacteria strain growth.

wilkesiana), were tested *in vitro* for anti-methicillin-resistant *Staphylococcus aureus* (MRSA) activity. Water and ethanol extracts of *T. avicennioides*, *P. discoideus*, *O. gratissimum*, and *A. wilkesiana* were both effective against MRSA. The ethanol extracts of these plants have MICs of 18.2 to 24.0 μg/mL and Minimum Bactericidal Concentrations (MBCs) of 30.4 to 37.0 μg/mL. In contrast, the MIC ranges for *B. ferruginea* and *A. conyzoides* ethanol and water extracts were 30.6 to 43.0 μg/mL as well as 55.4 to 71.0 μg/mL, respectively. The MBC values were higher in the two plants. The concentrations in this study were too high to be considered active. Anthraquinones were found in trace amounts in these four active plants [70].

Ethanol extracts of *Melianthus comosus*, *Melianthus major*, *Dodonaea viscosa* var. angustifolia, and *Withania somnifera* were found to be effective against both drug-sensitive and drug-resistant *S. aureus*. The minimum inhibitory concentrations for these plants ranged from 0.391 to 1.56 mg/mL. The XTT (2,3-Bis-(2-Methoxy-4-Nitro-5-Sulfophenyl)-*2H*-Tetrazolium-5-Carboxanilide) method was used to test the cytotoxicity of all these plants' ethyl alcohol extracts on Vero cells. *M. major* showed a 50% inhibitory activity (IC_{50}) of 52.76 g/mL and was therefore chosen for bioactive principle discovery. Two flavonoids were isolated from the leaves using column chromatography: quercetin 3-O-β-galactoside-6-gallate and kaempferol 3-O-α-arabinopyranoside. These molecules were discovered for the first time in this plant. These flavonoids also do not have antibacterial effect against the methicillin-sensitive strain of *S. aureus* at the highest concentration (500 g/mL). The antibacterial effect of *M. major* ethanolic extract observed in this research could be linked to the synergistic effects of the extract's quercetin 3-O-β-galactoside-6-gallate and kaempferol 3-O-α-arabinopyranoside and/or biomolecules not extracted in this study [71].

Five Nigerian plants mentioned as local antimicrobial agents, *Ocimum lamiifolium*, *Rosmarinus officinalis*, *Catharanthus roseus*, *Azadirachta indica*, as well as *Moringa stenopetala* [41, 72, 73], were evaluated *in vitro* against a panel of seven biofilm-forming MRSA. The medicinal plants' leaves extract, obtained by extraction with polar solvents of varying polarity, as well as the crude extracts had been evaluated for antimicrobial potential via well diffusion technique. The broth dilution method was employed to calculate the minimal inhibitory levels (MICs) and lowest bactericidal concentration levels (MBC) of extracts against MRSA. Furthermore, most efficacious plant extract was evaluated for anti-biofilm activity. Three of the five studied plants which displayed favorable antimicrobial property include *M. stenopetala*, *R. officinalis*, as well as *O. lamifolium*, according to the findings. Nonpolar solvents extracted antimicrobials effectively than organic solvents with medium and high polarity. This same crude ethanolic extract from *M. stenopetala* demonstrated the greatest range and rank of activity. Based on the MIC/MBC ratio, the ethanol extract of *M. stenopetala* had been found to be bacteriostatic. *M. stenopetala* extract strongly suppressed MRSA development inside the preformed biofilm matrix, according to the anti-biofilm assay [74].

Aspilia mossambicensis, *Ocimum gratissimum*, and *Toddalia asiatica* were identified and tested for bioactive antibacterial property. Hexane, ethyl acetate and methanol extract yields varied from 0.5% for *Ocimum gratissimum* stem bark ethyl acetate extract to 2.7% for *Toddalia asiatica* root bark methanolic extracts. The extracts were evaluated for *in vitro* experiments against Gram-positive-resistant *Staphylococcus aureus* (MRSA) using the disk diffusion method. Methanol extract of Asiatica stem bark had the maximum activity against methicillin-resistant *S. aureus* (15 mm diameter zone of inhibition). Preliminary phytochemical screening revealed the presence of the large percentage of alkaloids, polyphenols, steroids, and amines. By bioautographic selection, the organisms displayed antibacterial effect against methicillin-resistant *Staphylococcus aureus* (0.3125 mg/mL), which directly compared to the standard antibiotic gentamycin (0.5 mg/mL). These findings corroborate the ethno-medicinal utilization *Toddalia asiatica*, a Kenyan folkloric medicine, for bacterial-related conditions [75].

Sharquie et al. [76] studied the antibacterial effects of crude black tea (*Thea assamica*) treatments. Tea extracts were mixed into a 1% aqueous moisturizer (Group 1) and a 5% petroleum jelly base (Group 2), which were applied three to four times per day. Relieve rates in all these groups were compared to groups receiving framycetin as well as gramicidin cream (Group 3) or oral cefalixin (Group 4). The 5% green tea was just as efficacious as antibiotic treatments (cure rates of 81.3%, 72.2%, and 78.6% in groups 1–4, respectively). The cure rate in Group 1 was 37.5%. Regardless of the fact that sample size for this research seemed to be large, the number of patients in each treatment group was small. Furthermore, because the respondents were not designated randomly, this study was limited.

Another clinical study matched the administration of 4% tea tree oil (TTO) nasopharyngeal ointment and 5% TTO shower gel (intervention) to a conventional 2% mupirocin nasopharyngeal cream and triclosan body wash (routine) for the eradication of methicillin-resistant *Staphylococcus aureus* (MRSA). Thirty in-patients, contaminated or colonized with MRSA, were randomly assigned to receive TTO or conventional routine care for a maximum of 3 days. Infected patients received intravenous vancomycin as well, and then all participants were checked for MRSA carriage 48 as well as 96 hours after discontinuing topical treatment. Only 18 patients completed the trial. The intervention group cleared more infections than the healthy controls (5/8 versus 2/10). The intervention group included two patients who had been treated for 34 days: one managed to recover from the pathogen and the other patient remained chronically colonized. The group differences were not statistically relevant. This experiment was too small to yield a conclusive result [77].

4. Synergistic effect of synthetic and natural drugs for MRSA treatment

A novel strategy against antibiotic-resistant bacteria, such as MRSA, is synergistic or combination therapy. Plant extracts combined with common antibiotics show promising results in the treatment of MRSA infections. The microdilution method, also known as the checkerboard method, aids in determining the antibacterial interplay between natural and synthetic compounds. The synergistic combination of gentamycin and *C. esculenta* aqueous leaf extracts demonstrated antibacterial property against MRSA [78]. Blesson *et al.* [78] found that the phytochemicals in the leaf extracts bind to the MRSA cell wall and increase cell wall permeability as well as increasing the rate at which antibiotics enter MRSA. A synergistic relationship among *Alternathera brasiliensis* n-hexane fraction as well as erythromycin, ampicillin, and ciprofloxacin was also reported, with fractional inhibitory index (FIC) value varying from 0.208 to 0.375 [79]. Tomatidine, a steroidal alkaloid synthesized by solanaceous plants, possesses powerful and effective antibacterial properties against *S. aureus* either alone or in combination with aminoglycosides [80].

Piperine, biologically active substance present in pepper, has been shown to have excellent antibacterial properties against MRSA infections when combined with gentamycin [81]. Synergism, or the combination of drugs, is a novel concept in drug development and the treatment of drug-resistant bacteria. The combined action of drugs outperforms the individual actions of the medications. As a result, this method can be used to discover new and efficient drugs against resistant bacteria. In summary, herbal extracts combined with antibiotics such as quinolones, β-lactams, aminoglycosides, tetracyclines, and glycopeptides could greatly enhance antibacterial effects, reduce therapeutic dose, reduce adverse effects, and reverse MRSA resistance. As a result, botanicals coupled with antibiotics could be a beneficial MRSA treatment strategy [82].

5. Vaccines for MRSA treatment

MRSA's rising antibiotic resistance profile suggests that new interventions such as vaccines and antibiotics are required. There is precedent for developing effective and affordable bacterial vaccines, which aim at single antigens or toxins, specifically capsular polysaccharides. The implementation of these innovations to *S. aureus* is disrupted by the bacterium's complex pathogenic mechanisms. Because *S. aureus* can be found in the normal human flora, it has developed a variety of methods to colonize and evade host immune system, such as polymorphic expression of specific proteins and the release of redundant bacterial pathogens [83, 84]. Animal models, as well as *in vitro* and *ex vivo* models, are used in translational science studies to assess vaccine candidates' efficacy. Although several vaccine candidates demonstrated potential in preclinical testing in a variety of *in vivo* models, those that have advanced to late-stage drug trials have been unable to demonstrate efficacy in human trials [85, 86].

Two different vaccines were discovered [87]. StaphVAX is a bivalent polysaccharide and protein-conjugated vaccine that targets *S. aureus* capsular polysaccharide varieties 5 and 8 (CP5 and CP8) that are associated with roughly 80% of *S. aureus*. In two Phase III trials, the candidate was evaluated to avert bacteremia in end-stage renal dialysis victims during 3 to 54 weeks following immunization. Bacteremia was lowered by 57% during the initial 40 weeks, but potency declined to 26% during week 54 [88]. A conclusive Phase III study of 3600 hemodialysis patients evaluated for bacteremia found no significant difference between vaccinated and placebo controls. The vaccine-induced functional antibody titers throughout this second follow-up Phase III study are yet to be made public. The major reason for the failure of the second trial is currently being credited to production discrepancies among various vaccine lots used in the two trials [89]. Therefore, the candidate's development was halted. Another candidate, V710, induces immunity against the cell wall-anchored iron scavenger protein IsdB and was tested in a Phase III randomized controlled experiment involving approximately 8000 adults undergoing cardiac surgery. An interim analysis revealed a substantial increase in mortality caused by *S. aureus* infection, as well as a considerably higher level of other adverse effects [90].

Passive immunization strategies based on polyclonal as well as monoclonal antibodies (mAbs) were developed for individuals who are immunocompromised and unable to install an independent, robust immune response, as well as those who are at instantaneous threat of infection and do not have time for an active immunization to work properly. Five antibody candidates were already developed and tested in late-stage clinical trials, but none have shown efficacy [91].

Monoclonal antibodies, chemotherapy drugs, and centyrins are being designed in addition to bacteriophages. A number of these approaches have already been examined in humans, and the results have been promising. The attention has concentrated on developing a prophylactic product which might protect against potentially fatal *S. aureus* infections, although it is anticipated that such a vaccine will also protect against other S. aureus infections, including more frequently occurring infections of the skin and tissues [92–94].

Immune responses that safeguard against invasive *S. aureus* infections, along with host genetic factors as well as bacterial evasion mechanisms, are critical considerations for the continued development of safe and effective vaccines as well as immunotherapies against invasive *S. aureus* infections among humans [95]. Discussion on the significance of developing novel vaccine regimens that evoke effective cellular and humoral immune responses is common. This determines that enrolling vaccines in clinical trials provides the highest probability of success in addressing MRSA infections, and a better understanding of the synergy of immunotherapies, antibiotics, and vaccines could indeed aid in the design of future clinical trials [93].

6. Conclusion

Due to the poor prognosis and high cost of treatment associated with this infectious disease, MRSA infections are an increasing challenge for human society. Most antibiotics on the market are becoming less effective against bacterial resistance, particularly MRSA. Thus, new strategies for treating MRSA infections are required. Future MRSA infection treatment methods may include the following features: nanocarriers with a large surface area for targeted delivery of antibiotics with low inhibitory concentrations, design and implementation of antibody-based pharmacological agent therapies for the management of severe MRSA infections, multidrug approaches for handling drug-resistant pathogenic bacteria such as pharmaceutical chemicals, artificial and herbal drugs, and natural medicines, and breakage of MRSA biofilms using an appropriate targeting carrier system and biotic drugs.

Author details

Enitan Omobolanle Adesanya[1*] and Akingbolabo Daniel Ogunlakin[2]

1 Faculty of Pharmacy, Department of Pharmacognosy, Olabisi Onabanjo University, Ago Iwoye, Nigeria

2 Phytomedicine, Molecular Toxicology and Computational Biochemistry Research Group, Biochemistry Programmes, Bowen University, Iwo, Nigeria

*Address all correspondence to: enitadesanya@gmail.com

References

[1] Payne SC, Benninger MS. *Staphylococcus aureus* is a major pathogen in acute bacterial rhinosinusitis: A meta-analysis. Clinical Infectious Diseases. 2007;**45**(10):e121-e127

[2] Fisher B, Harvey RP, Champe PC. Lippincott's Illustrated Reviews: Microbiology. Lippincott's Illustrated Reviews. Hagerstown, Maryland: Lippincott Williams & Wilkins; 2007

[3] Crosby HA, Kwiecinski J, Horswill AR. *Staphylococcus aureus* aggregation and coagulation mechanisms, and their function in host–pathogen interactions. Advances in Applied Microbiology. 2016;**96**:1-41

[4] Staph Infection. 2021. https://www.nhs.uk/conditions/staphylococcal-infections. [Accessed: September 22, 2022]

[5] Lowy FD. Staphylococcal infections. In: Jameson J, Fauci AS, Kasper DL, Hauser SL, Longo DL, Loscalzo J, editors. Harrison's Principles of Internal Medicine. United States: McGraw Hill; 2018

[6] Alfatemi SM, Motamedifar M, Hadi N, Saraie HS. Analysis of virulence genes among methicillin resistant *Staphylococcus aureus* (MRSA) strains. Jundishapur journal of microbiology. 2014;7:e10741

[7] Marchione M. Dangerous staph germs found at West Coast beaches. 2009

[8] Tacconelli E, De Angelis G, Cataldo MA, Pozzi E, Cauda R. Does antibiotic exposure increase the risk of methicillin-resistant *Staphylococcus aureus* (MRSA) isolation? A systematic review and meta-analysis. The Journal of Antimicrobial Chemotherapy. 2008;**61**(1):26-38

[9] Li J, Jiang N, Ke Y, Feßler AT, Wang Y, Schwarz S, et al. Characterization of pig-associated methicillin-resistant *Staphylococcus aureus*. Veterinary Microbiology. 2017;**201**:183-187

[10] Markwart R, Willrich N, Eckmanns T, Werner G, Ayobami O. Low proportion of linezolid and daptomycin resistance among bloodborne vancomycin-resistant *Enterococcus faecium* and methicillin-resistant *Staphylococcus aureus* infections in Europe. Frontiers in Microbiology. 2021;**2021**:1379

[11] Pendleton JN, Gorman SP, Gilmore BF. Clinical relevance of the ESKAPE pathogens. Expert Review of Anti-Infective Therapy. 2013;**11**(3):297-308

[12] Chaudhary AS. A review of global initiatives to fight antibiotic resistance and recent antibiotics' discovery. Acta Pharmaceutica Sinica B. 2016;**6**(6):552-556

[13] Alekshun MN, Levy SB. Molecular mechanisms of antibacterial multidrug resistance. Cell. 2007;**128**(6):1037-1050

[14] Reygaert WC. An overview of the antimicrobial resistance mechanisms of bacteria. AIMS Microbiology. 2018;**4**(3):482-501

[15] Baker-Austin C, Wright MS, Stepanauskas R, McArthur JV. Co-selection of antibiotic and metal resistance. Trends in Microbiology. 2006;**14**(4):176-182

[16] Sarna LK, Wu N, Hwang SY, Siow YL, Karmin O. Berberine inhibits NADPH oxidase mediated superoxide anion production in macrophages. Canadian Journal of Physiology and Pharmacology. 2010;**88**(3):369-378

[17] Guo Y, Wang J, Niu G, Shui W, Sun Y, Zhou H, et al. A structural view of the antibiotic degradation enzyme NDM-1 from a superbug. Protein & Cell. 2011;**2**(5):384-394

[18] Karthikeyan K, Mark A, Timothy R, et al. Emergence of a new antibiotic resistance mechanism in India, Pakistan, and the UK: A molecular, biological, and epidemiological study. The Lancet Infectious Diseases. 2010;**10**(9):597-602

[19] Okwu MU, Olley M, Akpoka AO, Izevbuwa OE. Methicillin-resistant *Staphylococcus aureus* (MRSA) and anti-MRSA activities of extracts of some medicinal plants: A brief review. AIMS Microbiology. 2019;**5**(2):117

[20] Health Research and Educational Trust (HRET). Multidrug-resistant organisms. Infection change package. 2017. Available from: http://www.hrethiin.org. [Accessed: September 28, 2022]

[21] Johnson AP. Methicillin-resistant *Staphylococcus aureus*: The European landscape. Journal of Antimicrobial Chemotherapy. 2011;**66**(4):iv43-iv48

[22] Arunkumar V, Prabagaravarthanan R, Bhaskar M. Prevalence of Methicillin-resistant *Staphylococcus aureus* (MRSA) infections among patients admitted in critical care units in a tertiary care hospital. International Journal of Research and Medical Science. 2017;**5**:2362-2366

[23] Ravensbergen SJ, Berends M, Stienstra Y, Ott A. High prevalence of MRSA and ESBL among asylum seekers in the Netherlands. PLoS One. 2017;**12**(4):e0176481

[24] Sit PS, Teh CS, Idris N, Sam IC, Syed Omar SF, Sulaiman H, et al. Prevalence of Methicillin-resistant *Staphylococcus aureus* (MRSA) infection and the molecular characteristics of MRSA bacteremia over a two-year period in a tertiary teaching hospital in Malaysia. BMC Infectious Diseases. 2017;**17**:274

[25] Stefani S, Chung DR, Lindsay JA, Friedrich AW, Kearns AM, Westh H, et al. Meticillin-resistant *Staphylococcus aureus* (MRSA): Global epidemiology and harmonisation of typing methods. International Journal of Antimicrobial Agents. 2012;**39**(4):273-282

[26] Hamid V, Alijan T, Abdolvahab M, Ezzat AG. Evaluation of methicillin resistance *Staphylococcus aureus* isolated from patients in Golestan province-north of Iran. African Journal of Microbiology Research. 2011;**5**(4):432-436

[27] Akanbi BO, Mbe JU. Occurrence of methicillin and vancomycin resistant *Staphylococcus aureus* in University of Abuja Teaching Hospital, Abuja, Nigeria. African Journal of Clinical and Experimental Microbiology. 2013;**14**(1):10-13

[28] Goud R, Gupta S, Neogi U, Agarwal D, Naidu K, Chalannavar R, et al. Community prevalence of methicillin and vancomycin resistant *Staphylococcus aureus* in and around Bangalore, southern India. Revista da Sociedade Brasileira de Medicina Tropical. 2011;**44**:309-312

[29] Alo M, Ugah U, Okoro N. Epidemiology of vancomycin-resistant *Staphylococcus aureus* among clinical isolates in a tertiary hospital in Abakaliki, Nigeria. American Journal of Epidermiological Infectious Diseases. 2013;**1**:24-26

[30] Howden BP, Davies JK, Johnson PD, Stinear TP, Grayson ML. Reduced vancomycin susceptibility in *Staphylococcus aureus*, including vancomycin-intermediate and heterogeneous vancomycin-intermediate strains: Resistance mechanisms, laboratory detection, and clinical

implications. Clinical Microbiology Reviews. 2010;**23**(1):99-139

[31] Loomba PS, Taneja J, Mishra B. Methicillin and vancomycin resistant *S. aureus* in hospitalized patients. Journal of Global Infectious Diseases. 2010;**2**:275

[32] Cong Y, Yang S, Rao X. Vancomycin resistant *Staphylococcus aureus* infections: A review of case updating and clinical features. Journal of Advanced Research. 2020;**21**:169-176

[33] Hasan R, Acharjee M, Noor R. Prevalence of vancomycin resistant *Staphylococcus aureus* (VRSA) in methicillin resistant S. aureus (MRSA) strains isolated from burn wound infections. Tzu Chi Medical Journal. 2016;**28**(2):49-53

[34] Hernández-Aristizábal I, Ocampo-Ibáñez ID. Antimicrobial peptides with antibacterial activity against vancomycin-resistant *Staphylococcus aureus* strains: Classification, structures, and mechanisms of action. International Journal of Molecular Sciences. 2021;**22**(15):7927

[35] Gardete S, Tomasz A. Mechanisms of vancomycin resistance in *Staphylococcus aureus*. The Journal of Clinical Investigation. 2014;**124**(7):2836-2840

[36] Kali A. Antibiotics and bioactive natural products in treatment of methicillin resistant *Staphylococcus aureus*: A brief review. Pharmacognosy Reviews. 2015;**17**:29

[37] Kaur DC, Chate SS. Study of antibiotic resistance pattern in methicillin resistant *Staphylococcus aureus* with special reference to newer antibiotic. Journal of Global Infectious Diseases. 2015;7(2):78

[38] McGuinness WA, Malachowa N, DeLeo FR. Vancomycin Resistance in *Staphylococcus aureus*. The Yale Journal of Biology and Medicine. 2017;**90**:269-281

[39] Rodvold KA, McConeghy KW. Methicillin-resistant *Staphylococcus aureus* therapy: Past, present, and future. Clinical Infectious Diseases. 2014;**58**(1):S20-S27

[40] Subramani R, Narayanasamy M, Feussner KD. Plant-derived antimicrobials to fight against multi-drug-resistant human pathogens. Biotech. 2017;**7**(3):1-5

[41] Anyanwu MU, Okoye RC. Antimicrobial activity of Nigerian medicinal plants. Journal of Intercultural Ethnopharmacology. 2017;**6**(2):240

[42] World Health Organization (WHO). WHO publishes list of bacteria for which new antibiotics are urgently needed. 2017. Available from:http://who.int/mediacentre/news/releases/2017/bacteria-antibiotics. [Accessed September 21, 2022]

[43] Abouzeed YM, Elfahem A, Zgheel F, Ahmed MO. Antibacterial *in-vitro* activities of selected medicinal plants against methicillin resistant *Staphylococcus aureus* from Libyan environment. Journal of Environmental & Analytical Toxicology. 2013;**3**(6):1

[44] Fifendy M. Inhibitory power test of medicinal plants extract against bacterial growth methicillin resistant strains of *Staphylococcus aureus* (MRSA). In: Proceeding of International Conference on Research, Implementation and Education of Mathematics and Sciences 2014. Yogyakarta: Yogyakarta State University; 2014

[45] Sharma PU, Mack JP, Rojtman A. Ten highly effective essential oils inhibit growth of methicillin resistant *Staphylococcus aureus* (MRSA) and methicillin sensitive *Staphylococcus aureus* (MSSA). International Journal Pharmacy and Pharmacology. 2013;**5**:52-54

[46] Basri DF, Sandra V. Synergistic interaction of methanol extract from *Canarium odontophyllum* Miq. Leaf in combination with oxacillin against methicillin-resistant *Staphylococcus aureus* (MRSA) ATCC 33591. International Journal of Microbiology. 2016;**2016**:1-7

[47] Ansari M, Larijani K, Saber-Tehrani M. Antibacterial activity of Lippa citriodora herb essence against MRSA *Staphylococcus aureus*. African Journal of Microbiology Research. 2012;**6**(1):16-19

[48] Ansari MA, Alzohairy MA. One-pot facile green synthesis of silver nanoparticles using seed extract of Phoenix dactylifera and their bactericidal potential against MRSA. Evidence-Based Complementary and Alternative Medicine. 2018;**2018**:1-9

[49] Thompson DP. Inhibition of growth of *mycotoxigenic Fusarium* species by butylated hydroxyanisole and/or carvacrol. Journal of Food Protection. 1996;**59**(4):412-415

[50] Gurgel AP, da Silva JG, Grangeiro AR, Xavier HS, Oliveira RA, Pereira MS, et al. Antibacterial effects of Plectranthus amboinicus (Lour.) spreng (Lamiaceae) in methicillin resistant *Staphylococcus aureus* (MRSA). Latin American Journal of Pharmacy. 2009;**28**(3):460-464

[51] Ultee A, Gorris LGM, Smid EJ. Bactericidal activity of carvacrol towards the foodborne pathogen Bacillus cereus. Journal of Applied Microbiology. 1998;**85**:2111-2218

[52] Basri DF, Khairon R. Pharmacodynamic interaction of *Quercus infectoria* galls extract in combination with vancomycin against MRSA using microdilution checkerboard and time-kill assay. Evidence-based Complementary and Alternative Medicine. 2012;**2012**:1-6

[53] Baeshen MN, Al-Attas SG, Ahmed MM, Hanafy AA, Anwar Y, Alotibi IA, et al. The effect of Rhazya stricta aqueous leaves extract on MRSA genotypes in Jeddah province. Biotechnology and Biotechnological Equipment. 2016;**30**(2):368-374

[54] Caroline H, Graham M, David N, Linda MB, Colin EG, Paul JR, et al. Antibacterial activity of elder (Sambucus nigra L.) flower or berry against hospital pathogens. Journal of Medicinal Plants Research. 2010;**4**(17):1805-1809

[55] Chen D, Sun Z, Liu Y, Li Z, Liang H, Chen L, et al. Eleucanainones A and B: Two dimeric structures from the bulbs of *Eleutherine americana* with anti-MRSA activity. Organic Letters. 2020;**22**(9):3449-3453

[56] Manzuoerh R, Farahpour MR, Oryan A, Sonboli A. Effectiveness of topical administration of *Anethum graveolens* essential oil on MRSA-infected wounds. Biomedicine & Pharmacotherapy. 2019;**109**:1650-1658

[57] Abdallah EM. Antibacterial activity and toxicological studies on the oleo-gum resins of *Commiphora molmol* and *Boswellia papyrifera* [Doctoral dissertation, Ph. D thesis]. Faculty of Sci. and Technol. Al Neelain Univ. Sudan; 2009

[58] Voravuthikunchai SP, Kitpipit L. Activity of medicinal plant extracts against hospital isolates of methicillin-resistant *Staphylococcus aureus*. Clinical Microbiology and Infection. 2005b;**11**(6):510-512

[59] Gaur R, Gupta VK, Singh P, Pal A, Darokar MP, Bhakuni RS. Drug Resistance Reversal Potential of Isoliquiritigenin and Liquiritigenin Isolated from Glycyrrhiza glabra Against Methicillin-Resistant *Staphylococcus aureus* (MRSA). Phytotherapy Research. 2016;**30**(10):1708-1715

[60] Arshad N, Mehreen A, Liaqat I, Arshad M, Afrasiab H. *In vivo* screening and evaluation of four herbs against MRSA infections. BMC Complementary and Alternative Medicine. 2017;**17**(1):1-7

[61] Hemaiswarya S, Kruthiventi AK, Doble M. Synergism between natural products and antibiotics against infectious diseases. Phytomedicine. 2008;**15**(8):639-652

[62] Van Vuuren SF. Antimicrobial activity of South African medicinal plants. Journal of Ethnopharmacology. 2008;**119**(3):462-472

[63] Chew YL, Ling Chan EW, Tan PL, Lim YY, Stanslas J, Goh JK. Assessment of phytochemical content, polyphenolic composition, antioxidant and antibacterial activities of Leguminosae medicinal plants in Peninsular Malaysia. BMC Complementary and Alternative Medicine. 2011;**11**(1):1

[64] Lapornik B, Prošek M, Wondra AG. Comparison of extracts prepared from plant by-products using different solvents and extraction time. Journal of Food Engineering. 2005;**71**(2):214-222

[65] Tiwari P, Kumar B, Kaur M, Kaur G, Kaur H. Phytochemical screening and extraction: A review. Internationale pharmaceutica sciencia. 2011;**1**(1):98-106

[66] Akinjogunla OJ, Yah CS, Eghafona NO, Ogbemudia FO. Antibacterial activity of leave extracts of Nymphaea lotus (Nymphaeaceae) on methicillin *resistant Staphylococcus aureus* (MRSA) and vancomycin resistant *Staphylococcus aureus* (VRSA) isolated from clinical samples. Annals of Biological Research. 2010;**1**(2):174-184

[67] Aliyu AB, Musa AM, Abdullahi MS, Oyewale AO, Gwarzo US. Activity of plant extracts used in northern Nigerian traditional medicine against methicillin-resistant *Staphylococcus aureus* (MRSA). Nigerian Journal of Pharmaceutical Sciences. 2008;**7**(1):1-8

[68] Cowan MM. Plant products as antimicrobial agents. Clinical Microbiology Reviews. 1999;**12**(4):564-582

[69] Wikaningtyas P, Sukandar EY. The antibacterial activity of selected plants towards resistant bacteria isolated from clinical specimens. Asian Pacific Journal of Tropical Biomedicine. 2016;**6**(1):16-19

[70] Akinyemi KO, Oladapo O, Okwara CE, Ibe CC, Fasure KA. Screening of crude extracts of six medicinal plants used in South-West Nigerian unorthodox medicine for anti-methicillin resistant *Staphylococcus aureus* activity. BMC Complementary and Alternative Medicine. 2005;**5**(1):1-7

[71] Heyman HM, Hussein AA, Meyer JJ, Lall N. Antibacterial activity of South African medicinal plants against methicillin resistant *Staphylococcus aureus*. Pharmaceutical Biology. 2009;**47**(1):67-71

[72] Bello OM, Ibitoye T, Adetunji C. Assessing antimicrobial agents of Nigeria flora. Journal of King Saud University-Science. 2019;**31**(4):1379-1383

[73] Ugboko HU, Nwinyi OC, Oranusi SU, Fatoki TH, Omonhinmin CA. Antimicrobial importance of medicinal plants in Nigeria. The Scientific World Journal. 2020;**2020**:7059323

[74] Manilal A, Sabu KR, Shewangizaw M, Aklilu A, Seid M, Merdekios B, et al. *In vitro* antibacterial activity of medicinal plants against biofilm-forming methicillin-resistant *Staphylococcus aureus*: Efficacy of *Moringa stenopetala* and *Rosmarinus officinalis* extracts. Heliyon. 2020;**6**(1):e03303

[75] Munyendo WL, Orwa JA, Rukunga GM, Bii CC. Bacteriostatic and bactericidal activities of *Aspilia mossambicensis*, *Ocimum gratissimum* and *Toddalia asiatica* extracts on selected pathogenic bacteria. Research Journal of Medical Plant. 2011;**5**(6):717-727

[76] Sharquie KE, Turfi IA, Salloum SM. The antibacterial activity of tea *in vitro* and *in vivo* (in patients with impetigo contagiosa). The Journal of Dermatology. 2000;**27**(11):706-710

[77] Caelli M, Porteous J, Carson CF, Heller R, Riley TV. Tea tree oil as an alternative topical decolonization agent for methicillin-resistant *Staphylococcus aureus*. International Journal of Aromatherapy. 2001;**11**(2):97-99

[78] Blesson J, Saji CV, Nivya RM, Kumar R. Synergistic antibacterial activity of natural plant extracts and antibiotics against methicillin resistant *Staphylococcus aureus* (MRSA). World Journal of Pharmacy and Pharmaceutical Sciences. 2015;**4**(3):741-763

[79] Adesanya EO, Sonibare MA, Ajaiyeoba EO, Egieyeh SA. Compounds isolated from hexane fraction of *Alternanthera brasiliensis* show synergistic activity against methicillin resistant *Staphylococcus aureus*. Pharmaceutical Applications. 2021;**1**(1):123-146

[80] Jiang QW, Chen MW, Cheng KJ, Yu PZ, Wei X, Shi Z. Therapeutic potential of steroidal alkaloids in cancer and other diseases. Medicinal Research Reviews. 2016;**36**(1):119-143

[81] Khameneh B, Iranshahy M, Ghandadi M, Ghoochi Atashbeyk D, Fazly Bazzaz BS, Iranshahi M. Investigation of the antibacterial activity and efflux pump inhibitory effect of co-loaded piperine and gentamicin nanoliposomes in methicillin-resistant *Staphylococcus aureus*. Drug Development and Industrial Pharmacy. 2015;**41**(6):989-994

[82] Bao M, Zhang L, Liu B, Li L, Zhang Y, Zhao H, et al. Synergistic effects of anti-MRSA herbal extracts combined with antibiotics. Future Microbiology. 2020;**15**(13):1265-1276

[83] Dreisbach A, van Dijl JM, Buist G. The cell surface proteome of *Staphylococcus aureus*. Proteomics. 2011;**11**(15):3154-3168

[84] Golubchik T, Batty EM, Miller RR, Farr H, Young BC, Larner-Svensson H, Fung R, Godwin H, Knox K, Votintseva A, Everitt RG. Within-host evolution of *Staphylococcus aureus* during asymptomatic carriage. PloS ONE. 2013;**8**(5):e61319

[85] Verkaik NJ, Van Wamel WJ, Van Belkum A. Immunotherapeutic approaches against *Staphylococcus aureus*. Immunotherapy. 2011;**3**(9):1063-1073

[86] Salgado-Pabón W, Schlievert PM. Models matter: The search for an effective *Staphylococcus aureus* vaccine. Nature Reviews Microbiology. 2014;**12**(8):585-591

[87] Schaffer AC, Lee JC. Vaccination and passive immunisation against *Staphylococcus aureus*. International Journal of Antimicrobial Agents. 2008 Nov 1;**32**:S71-S78

[88] Fattom AI, Horwith G, Fuller S, Propst M, Naso R. Development of StaphVAX™, a polysaccharide conjugate vaccine against *S. aureus* infection: From the lab bench to phase III clinical trials. Vaccine. 2004;**22**(7):880-887

[89] Fattom A, Matalon A, Buerkert J, Taylor K, Damaso S, Boutriau D. Efficacy profile of a bivalent *Staphylococcus*

aureus glycoconjugated vaccine in adults on hemodialysis: Phase III randomized study. Human Vaccines & Immunotherapeutics. 2015;**11**(3):632-641

[90] Fowler VG, Allen KB, Moreira ED, Moustafa M, Isgro F, Boucher HW, et al. Effect of an investigational vaccine for preventing *Staphylococcus aureus* infections after cardiothoracic surgery: A randomized trial. Journal of the American Medical Association. 2013;**309**(13):1368-1378

[91] Fowler VG Jr, Proctor RA. Where does a *Staphylococcus aureus* vaccine stand? Clinical Microbiology and Infection. 2014:66-75

[92] Bagnoli F. *Staphylococcus aureus* toxin antibodies: Good companions of antibiotics and vaccines. Virulence. 2017;**8**(7):1037-1042

[93] Clegg J, Soldaini E, McLoughlin RM, Rittenhouse S, Bagnoli F, Phogat S. *Staphylococcus aureus* vaccine research and development: The past, present and future, including novel therapeutic strategies. Frontiers in Immunology. 2021;**2021**:2693

[94] Nandhini P, Kumar P, Mickymaray S, Alothaim AS, Somasundaram J, Rajan M. Recent developments in methicillin-resistant *Staphylococcus aureus* (MRSA) treatment: A review. Antibiotics. 2022;**11**(5):606

[95] Miller LS, Fowler VG Jr, Shukla SK, Rose WE, Proctor RA. Development of a vaccine against *Staphylococcus aureus* invasive infections: Evidence based on human immunity, genetics and bacterial evasion mechanisms. FEMS Microbiology Reviews. 2020;**44**(1):123-153